I0839940

THE RETRO-SURVIVALIST

HANDBOOK – REV-2

TAKING CONTROL of your LIFE

One step at a Time!

By

Donald W Bobbitt

ISBN-10: 1984365843
ISBN-13: 978-1984365842

DISCLAIMER

The information provided in this book is true and accurate as far as the author is aware at the time the information in this book was compiled. Care was taken to research everything presented here, on the web, utilizing what were assumed to be reliable sources. But if there are any errors present in this book, the author cannot be held responsible for accuracy of the information presented here nor for any damage, injury or problems incurred by or to the reader or any others.

The author assumes that the reader always follows proper safety procedures when managing their health and their lifestyle and the author cannot be held responsible in any way for any damages, injuries or problems encountered by the reader, under any circumstances.

Any Characters and Events in this book are fictitious. Any similarities to real persons, living or dead, is coincidental, and not intended by the Author.

DEDICATION

This book is dedicated to the patience of my wife, Helen, who has spent countless hours alone while I worked on the construction of this Book.

Table of Contents

The RETRO-SURVIVALIST

BOOK-1 – STEPS to Taking Control

This book is designed to be a quick reference for those people who are interested in "going RETRO" where it is logical to get their bodies and lives under their control by using old-fashioned, tried and true methods of living where it makes sense for them.

I call these people **Retro-Survivalists**.

So what is a Retro-Survivalist?

A Retro-Survivalist is someone who feels that there must be; healthier, cheaper and safer ways to do things in this modern world of ours than what is thrust at us by the big corporations of the world.

Retro-Survivalists also believe that even though we Americans have a longer life expectancy than ever, we are literally inundated, every day of our lives, with products that are loaded with strange chemicals and additives.

We feel that our bodies should not be subjected to such modified and polluted foods in our stores nor by medicines with ingredients that have so many dangerous side effects, just so the; growers, producers and packers can make even larger profits off of us.

A Retro-Survivalist is someone who believes that at least some of our day-to-day methods of living and taking care of our bodies were once done simpler and cheaper. We know that many health treatments popular with our ancestors are probably still applicable today, if we only knew what they were and how they were done.

We're tired of **being misled by advertisers** and we want to be told exactly what we are being fed and treated with. We not only want to know what the corporations are putting into our foods and medications, but we also want to know about other healthier options used in the past should once again be available for us to choose from.

We want clearly defined options that we can select from and information that clearly explains any potential health risks associated with our selection's options.

Donald W Bobbitt

We should have more, naturally grown, processed and packaged foods on our supermarket shelves. We want access to safer methods to not only grow and prepare our own foods but also methods for treating the simpler human illnesses, just as our forebears did.

Many of the new pharmaceutical drugs and their ingredients are introduced to the public as being wonders of science, at first, only to be shown to have disastrous side effects when used over a long period of time.

Of course, most of us want to enjoy our modern conveniences, especially when it comes to foods and medicines. But shouldn't we also have access to the choices that are often safer, more natural and healthier for ourselves and our children?

And if the big pharmaceutical corporations will not be proactive and make the nation's health their top priority, then we should have access to the knowledge of how to grow our own, healthier foods in some limited manner where we control the process and ingredients ourselves or at least purchase these more natural products.

Take Control of what you can

This book is focused on helping the reader **TAKE CONTROL** of many of the day-to-day things they use in their lives, from what to eat to how to treat the more common illnesses they may contract.

This book is not designed to teach you how to just "go off of the Grid" and immediately start living your own self-sustained lifestyle.

Instead it is designed to provide pieces of information and ideas that can help you understand how to buy safer and healthier foods, how to grow some of your own foods, and how to make yourself and your family more self-sufficient and healthy.

Simply use the **Table of Contents** and the **Index** to get to the appropriate section that interests you.

ORGANIC, NATURAL or MYSTERY FOODS?

In today's world of industrialized food production the consumer is at the mercy of the producers when it comes to how the food or meat is grown and what chemicals can be used in its production.

Pick up a can of beans or grab a bag of chips or crackers and you quickly realize that you need to be a chemist to figure out what some of the ingredients are and what they are doing in your food.

Add to this the fact that our meats can be fed so many different chemicals that are not even on any label and you can understandably start to worry about what is safe and what is not.

There are essentially three general categories that you can place your foods if you are concerned about your family's health, and these are Organic Foods, Natural Foods and what I call Mystery Foods.

Organic Foods

The U.S. Department of Agriculture or USDA regulates the standard for organically grown foods, and how they are labeled.

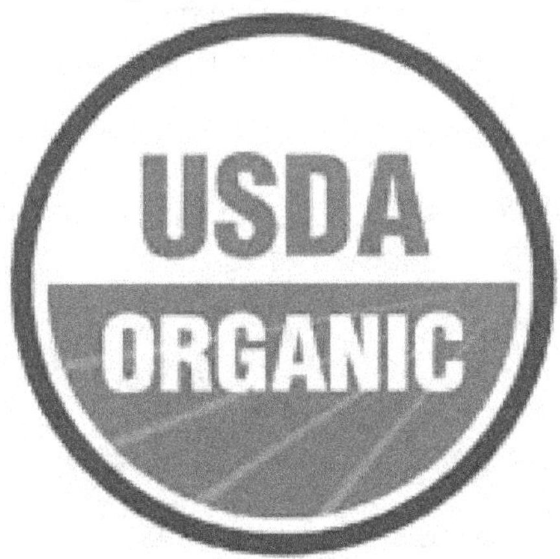

There are strict standards that regulate not only how these foods are grown but also how they are handled and processed.

The small farmer who produces and sells less than $5000 in organic foods a year are exempt from government certification but at the same time they are required to follow all of the USDA standards for the production of organic foods.

There are three labels that certified organic food producers could use on their products. You should look for the USDA ORGANIC label itself, along with one of the three following phrases; **100% Organic** or **Organic**, or **Made with Organic ingredients**.

The USDA defines and inspects these foods to be within their guidelines, which are:

- 100% Organic labeled foods must be 100% organic or made for 100% organic ingredients.
- Organic labeled foods must be at least 95%, or more, organic or must be made of 95% or more organic ingredients.
- Made with Organic labeled foods must be at least 70% or more organic or must be made with 70% or more organic ingredients. These foods can use this label but they cannot carry the USDA organic label
- Foods that are less than 70% organic cannot use the word organic on their labels in any way even if they do include some organic ingredients.

Organic foods contain significantly less pesticides than their non-organic counterparts according to the USDA and thus pose less health risks for the consumer.

Read the labels, even on the Organic foods. The organic label does not mean that the food is more nutritious, only that it was raised or grown to federal organic food standards.

Organic foods can still be loaded with salt sugar, fats and calories.

Natural Foods

Presently there is no formal definition of the term **Natural Food** by the Food and Drug Administration. The definition of Natural that is presently used in food labeling is presently arbitrarily defined by each particular manufacturer or industry sector and not necessarily a generic one that the consumer can trust.

To date, the FDA has not objected to the different food industries using the term as a statement that their food does not contain such things as artificial flavors, added colors or other synthetic substances.

So, although there is no official definition of what the terms **Natural** and **Natural Food** really means the use of these terms on food labels by their producers implies that the food product is minimally processed and does not contain manufactured ingredients such as sweeteners, flavorings, food colorings or hormones.

On a positive note, even though neither the USDA nor the FDA have rules for "**Natural Foods**" the Food, Drug and Cosmetic Act prohibits any labeling that is false or misleading.

Because of this unregulated category of foods, the consumer should be very cautious when they see a food labeled as either being Natural or being a Natural Food.

Mystery Foods

I call these other foods **Mystery Foods,** not because they are totally uncontrolled or even unsafe, but because the federal laws and controls applied to these other foods are a mystery to the common consumer.

Literally every category of foods that are consumed in America has different constraints on the growers and processors as to approved additives, preservatives and other chemicals that can be used.

And, the individual grower's lobbyists in Congress are constantly working to change these constraints. The result is that we are now consuming some foods which are full of chemicals that were added to benefit the manufacturer and not for the good of the consumer.

FOOD Ingredients Labels

Always read the labels on packaged foods you purchase. There is a wealth of information available to the consumer on the label of all packaged foods for you to check out.

Read the chapter called **Understanding Food Labels** for a good explanation of what you are eating and as a tool for brand comparisons.

FOOD Safety Tips

Here are some tips that the consumer can follow in order to insure they are purchasing healthier foods.

- When they are in season, purchase your fruits and vegetables at roadside markets when possible.
- Always asl your local grocer, especially the large chain stores where their fresh vegetables and fruits are grown. Many are imported from other countries.
- Always wash and scrub whatever you purchase to remove as much dirt, bacteria, pesticides and processing residue as possible before cooking or consuming them.
- Read the labels and check if the fruits and vegetables are imported from other countries. Presently over 60% of fresh vegetables and fruits consumed in the US are imported from other countries.
- These countries are required to comply with FDA regulations for growing and processing what they ship to the US, just as American producers do. But keep in mind that the agency's inspection staffs for overseas producers are notoriously sparse.

UNDERSTANDING FOOD FRESHNESS and LABELS

In our modern world, if you are concerned about what you and your family are eating then your first step to becoming knowledgeable is for you to read the labels on those cans and bags of foods you purchase very closely.

Once you pick up a can of your favorite beans or a bag of potato chips, and actually read the labels you will have opened up a new world of valuable (and sometimes scary) information.

NUTRITION Information

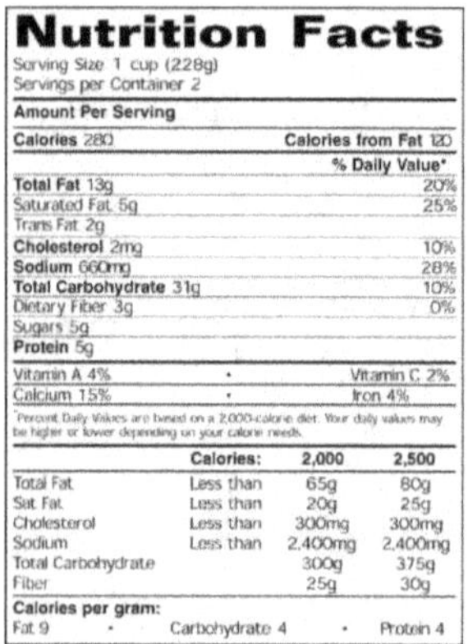

The USDA requires the listing of the nutritional information of a packaged food. It will include the percentage of the official **Minimum Daily Requirement (MDR)** that is based on a 2000 calories a day diet.

The nutritional data table will include such data as serving size; servings per container, and then for each serving it will list percentage of the MDR of Fats, Total Fats, Saturated Fats, and Trans Fats.

It also lists the percentage of the other nutrients such as Cholesterol, Carbohydrates, Sodium, Protein, Salt, Sugar, Calcium, Dietary Fiber and Iron as well as any Vitamins present.

Using this nutritional data can help you select healthier food options and select your foods for a better diet.

FOOD Ingredients

When you find the Ingredients listing the first thing you should notice is the order of the ingredients.

The ingredients should be listed in the order of their volume, so there is more of the first ingredient than there is of the second, and more of the second than of the third, and so on down the list.

The next thing you will notice is that there are some ingredients that have chemical sounding names.

These are the ones you need to know about because they are usually added for different reasons but most are added as preservatives or for other processing or growth purposes.

GMO – Genetically Modified Organism

The business of genetically modifying foods has drawn criticism for decades and still there is no clear-cut data that can totally condemn this practice. Agri-Business is the largest proponent of GMO's as they focus on changes that allow for larger production volumes of certain foods.

On the other side of the fence are the people who can show that, unchecked; many of these modified foods have been proven as being dangerous to the health of the consumer. More and more of us will need to take a position as this practice expands around the world.

So many packaged foods today can include GMO foods and ingredients that everyone needs to recognize the keywords on labels that indicate you are looking at a food that is itself a genetically modified organism or has GMO ingredients.

The major crops that are genetically modified and sold on the market today are; **Canola, Corn, Cottonseed** and **Soy,** and of course, the oils made from these modified foods. Presently, if you are concerned about GMO's then you are safer using unmodified versions of **Olive, Safflower** and **Sunflower Oils**, as corporations have not started producing any modified versions of them to date.

Here are just a few of the keywords you should question when you will find them on the labels of many GMO foods:

Amino Acids, Ascorbic Acid, Aspartame, Citric Acid, Emulsified, Emulsifiers, "from concentrate", Fructose, Hydrolyzed Vegetable Protein, Lactic Acid, Maltodestrins, Modified Corn, Modified Soy and MSG (Monosodium Glutamate).

OTHER ECO-FRIENDLY LABELS

With the growing public concerns over the misrepresentation of processed foods and their contents, a number of organizations have sprung up with their own label keywords.

These keywords are used by these organizations to represent or attempt to represent the safety of their products. But, often, these corporations and their labeling often just add to the confusion about the products and whether they are actually better or safer for humans.

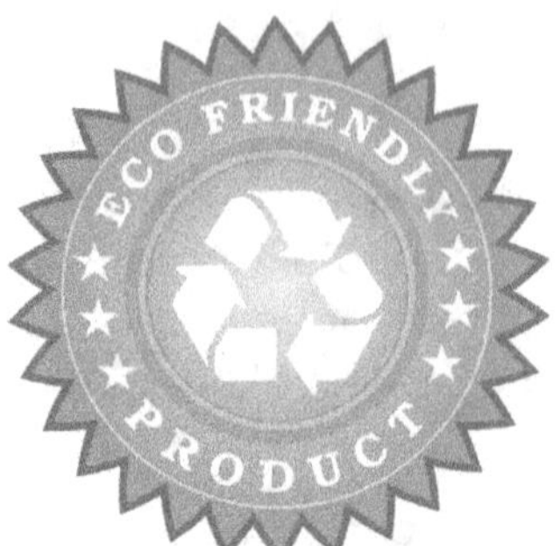

On the positive side, there is one popular perspective we the consumer can rely on. We can keep in mind when we read these supposed Eco-Friendly labels that, in the US, we do have our **Federal "Truth in Labeling" laws that override any attempts at giving the public false information**.

And, we at least know that, these corporations are aware of their liability when they define these specialized food label keywords.

Some of these companies using Eco-Friendly labels, for instance when using a word like "Organic", are certified by a third-party testing organization to comply with certain requirements such as the labeling of meats by the USDA. The USDA does provide a well regulated monitoring and testing system that the public has come to trust and rely on for meats.

But, remember, the use of some of these newer "label keywords" are well managed while there are some which are not so well managed at all. The onus is on the public to research and understand these companies and their standards.

Some of these self-regulated companies may meet the letter of the law with their standards and presentation of their testing methodology and resultant data, but they can also tend to exaggerate or even mislead the public with the vagueness of their labeling.

Review **Table B2-2** for a list of just a few of these labels that are commonly used with a short definition of each.

PLUS CODES

I am sure that you have noticed those little nuisance stickers on your fresh fruits and vegetables. You know that little round sticker on every Apple you pick up to eat that is impossible to remove?

Well if you look closer, you will see that the stickers have a number code on them.

These code numbers are managed by an organization, PLU that defines the code meaning.

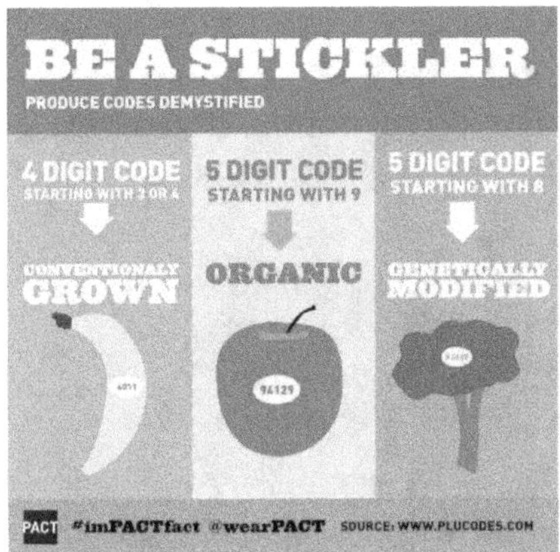

When you are selecting produce in your supermarket, be sure to examine the sticker and look at the first digit number.

The first digit number defines the fruit as shown in this chart. But you should also know that GMO products are not required to be labeled as such.

A Label Reading Experiment by the Author

Even though my wife and I do try to "eat smart" we often need to work very hard to know what we are putting into our bodies. To show you, I decided to run a small experiment.

So, I walked over to our pantry and arbitrarily took out four items to run my little experiment on: a can of red beans, a can of olives, a jar of peanut butter and a can of soup.

After reading the label of each can here are some of the chemicals listed on the labels that I realized I had no idea what they were:

Peanut Butter; fully hydrogenated oil (rapeseed or soybean), mono and glycerides

Olives; ferrous gluconate (to stabilize color)

Chicken Tuscany Soup; Corn Protein (hydrolyzed), Potassium Chloride, Maltodextrine, Isolate, Sodium Phosphate, Natural Flavor, Calcium Chloride, Beta Carotene (color)

Red Beans; No Ingredients were listed?

So what did I find in my little experiment?

Well, first of all, when I see hydrogenated oil, I know that this means the food has Trans Fats and I try to not eat much of this deadly food additive at all, and as to **Rapeseed Oil**? I do know that the FDA has a limit on how much of this potentially toxic chemical is allowed in foods in the US.

Also, I have a slight allergy to foods with MSG (monosodium glutamate) in them, so I do try to avoid foods with this additive in them.

Next, I had to ask myself, just what is **natural flavor** and why do canned black olives need a chemical to stabilize the color? Natural Flavor was one ingredient I couldn't find a reference to, at all, even on the web.

As to the other additives, when I looked them up I realized I was in a world of chemical definitions that I will not attempt to share here. But, after reading the listing of ingredients I am now wary of as simple as my canned soup.

Are these additives safe for me? I don't know, really, and honestly I and other average Americans rarely take the time to research such complicated names.

But, when I do look one up, it is a rare instance that I have found one that is considered totally safe or good for me.

It is a personal battle of mine to read these package labels and at least attempt to keep as many of such additives with their strange names to a minimum in my foods.

You should ask yourself; what's sitting in your pantry?

Understanding Food Freshness

Many of the foods you see in supermarkets do not just "go bad" on their labeled "sell by date". In fact, these dates are set as guidelines for the store itself and often just to provide a reference for the customer.

Even though the "sell by date" is important and should be checked on all food purchases, there is still some room for you to take advantage of those sale items that have dates that expire soon.

And, some foods are not labeled with "sell by dates" at all. But there are some standards you can follow with these foods to assure you are still managing your older foods properly.

Following are some facts you can use when handling your stored foods or reading those Sell By dates on your food labels:

Cheeses

Cheeses can still be good for as long as three to four months after their "sell by date". The hard varieties will last even longer because they contain less moisture for bacteria's and fungi to grow on.

Good cheeses are expensive and when you have leftover portions seal them tightly in plastic wrap with a minimal amount of air in the package to avoid growing mold. Also, if you check and your cheese had some mold on it, cut away the portions with the mold and the cheese will still be useable.

Eggs

Eggs, when kept on a shelf in the fridge and in their original containers can easily remain useable for three or four weeks past their labeled **"Sell By date"**. And, of course, when you can, cook those older eggs first.

Herbs and Spices

Dried, ground or packaged Herbs and Spices once they have been opened will still be OK for up to six months, but you should toss them if they "lose their zest".

Just take a sniff and maybe take a small taste to make up your mind about their freshness.

Whole Spices, if stored tightly in a container can still be good for use for up to two years.

Meats

Raw Meats such as steaks, chops and roasts can be stored in the freezer for up to 12 months if they are packaged and sealed properly. Ground meats should be used within 4 months and cooked meats can be kept frozen for up to 4 months before they begin losing their favor.

Milk

Milk will still be good up to a week past its "sell by date" on its label. But remember, it must be stored at a 40F or lower temperature.

Store it in the back of your fridge to keep it away from those warmer temperatures when you open your fridge door.

Oils

Oils used for cooking such as Vegetable or Olive Oil are good for up to six months after they are opened. Many are still useable longer but should be checked for such things as the growth of molds or discoloration.

Pasta

Packaged Pasta is still useable for a year or longer when stored in the pantry, but after that you should consider tossing it.

Processed Meats

Processed Meats or lunchmeats can last three to five days beyond their "sell by date". When it's stored in a sealed plastic package the meat may be good even longer. They should be stored in the meat drawer of your fridge because this will keep the cold air in when the fridge is opened.

If the package is opened, and the meat has a slimy film and an unpleasant odor, then you should toss it.

Rice

Packaged Rice, like pasta, is still useable for a year or longer when properly stored in the pantry. After that, you should consider toss it.

Sugar

Packaged Sugar, like pasta and rice, is still useable for a year or longer when stored properly in your pantry. Some people recommend that you should consider tossing it if it has been stored for such a long time.

Yogurt

Yogurt can be kept as long as two weeks past its "sell by date" if it is stored in a cold fridge. When you open your yogurt, check that it doesn't have any mold or possibly a bad odor. If so, then toss it.

But, if your yogurt has separated and has water on top, when you open it, this is normal and you just need to stir it well and blend it back to its original consistency.

When storing foods, any foods, seal them properly and keep as much air as you can away from them.

SUPERMARKETS and THEIR PRIORITIES

Supermarkets! Those places that the vast majority of us shop at for our food do not exist just for our convenience. In fact, the customer must realize that a major corporation owns the neighborhood supermarket and that they are there to make a profit, not friends.

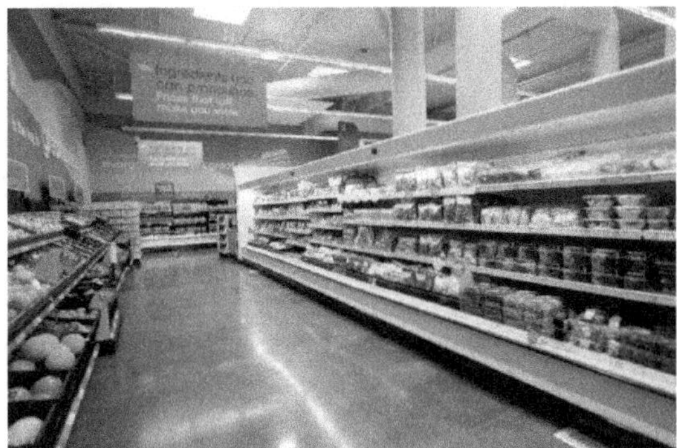

The corporations that own the major supermarkets in our country locate their retail food stores strategically for certain specific population groups.

You must already have noticed that a supermarket in an area that the majority of the population is poor will be smaller and have a much more limited variety of foods available than one that is in an area with a predominately middle class demographic.

And, in the same vein, a supermarket in a middle class area will not provide the variety and selection of foods that one that has residents who are higher paid professionals.

Supermarkets for the Poor

A supermarket in a poor area of a city will have a majority of its offered products that are fast foods, easy to prepare foods and less nutritious foods overall. They will have a very small selection of fresh foods, if any at all.

And, the aisles will be narrow and crowded to maximize the offerings they do provide.

Most meats and cheeses in these stores will often be pre-packaged and frozen at other sites in what they consider affordable sizes. The store will have a small butcher section, if any at all, because meats have a very short shelf life and if very few people in the poorer areas can afford fresh meats, then why offer such options to them.

You will often find a freezer selection of frozen meats that obviously can be kept available longer. The selection of dairy products and canned goods will be just as restricted and offering mostly basic canned beans and vegetables that happen to be more affordable.

Their priority when providing foods for areas with poorer demographics is to stock cheap and basic foods, not luxury or imported foods.

Supermarkets for the Middle Class

A supermarket in a middle class area will usually provide a very good selection of fresh vegetables and fruits, a wide selection of deli meats, and probably a small bakery of fresh breads and cakes.

This is in addition to better meats, cheeses, and other dairy products along with a wider selection of canned goods, cereals and snacks.

Supermarkets for the Upper Middle Class

Of course the trend continues when you walk into a supermarket that is in an area where professionals and other well-to-do customers shop. Their supermarkets will be very large, have wide and well-lit aisles and wide selections of food options in literally every section.

They will often also have such luxury sections as; olive bars, fresh prepared entrees and side dishes for the consumer to take home, large wine selections, imported cheeses, large selections of fresh baked goods, and much more.

Shopping in these high-end supermarkets is both a delight, while shopping, as well as a pain in your wallet, when you check out and see your bill.

Those specialty and imported items are not only expensive, generally, but the corporations know that their customers make more money and thus will bear with a little more of a profit margin for the convenience provided.

Supermarket Layouts push foods

When you walk into the front door of a supermarket, you are immediately assailed with a series of subtle but impressive marketing tricks designed to take your money.

You go to a typical supermarket and enter the front door, grab a shopping cart and right beside the carts there will be a shopping flyer which lists the items that they want really you to purchase, while there.

Discounts and Coupons

Some items in the flyer will be listed and described with colorful pictures and text, while other items will be offered at a discount or there might even be a coupon in the flyer for the shopper to use.

Don't be mistaken, these items are what the store wants you to buy and buy now. They want you to think; Wow, I can get a dollar off of that large bottle of product-X, I had better get that while it is so cheap.

In reality, the price has been lowered for one of several reasons. One reason might be that the manufacturer of the product has too much inventory of product-X in their warehouse and they are willing to offer a one-dollar discount via a coupon or discount at the cash register to lower their inventory.

The product may be even seasonal and they may just want to clear their warehouses of the product to make room for another product that they produce.

Or, possibly, the retailer is pushing them to get their product off of their shelves because it is not moving at the retail price.

There are a lot of reasons why they are offering discounts on supermarket products, but these discounts are offered for financial reasons and not as you might think for your convenience.

Meats and Fresh Foods

You need to understand that meats and fresh foods are perishable and have a very limited shelf life.

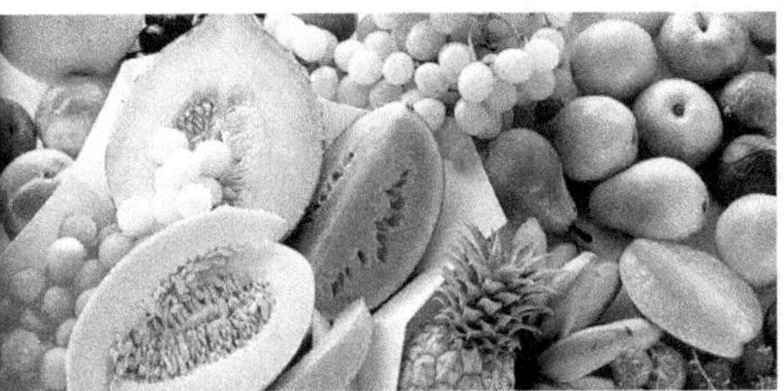

Because of this fact, the supermarkets want these foods to move off of their shelves as quickly as possible.

Here are a few facts and tips for you to be aware of when you are selecting from these initial offerings in the store.

Fresh fruits and vegetables that are laid out individually for you to select from will be the premium and freshest that they have to sell. If you look carefully, there will also be pre-packaged fruits and vegetables displayed for you to select from.

These packaged foods can often be less fresh than you might expect and some will even be on the verge of being bad.

Who hasn't picked up a sealed package of strawberries or cherry tomatoes or other supposedly fresh goods only to find that several of the ones at the bottom of the package are already crushed or even rotten?

And who hasn't picked up a bag of lemons or oranges and even though they may be smaller than what is displayed individually, they are so cheap that you go ahead and buy the bag? Also who, when they makes this decision to buy the cheap bag because of the price, hasn't found at least one or two items in the bag that are bad or damaged product?

Now we get to the meats. There are certain FDA standards on the definitions of meat categories and even some on the expiration dates for meats.

When meats are cut and placed on display they will have a **"sell by date"** shown on the label.

This end date is actually just a guideline and does not really indicate that the meat is bad, only that it is possibly no longer in its best condition.

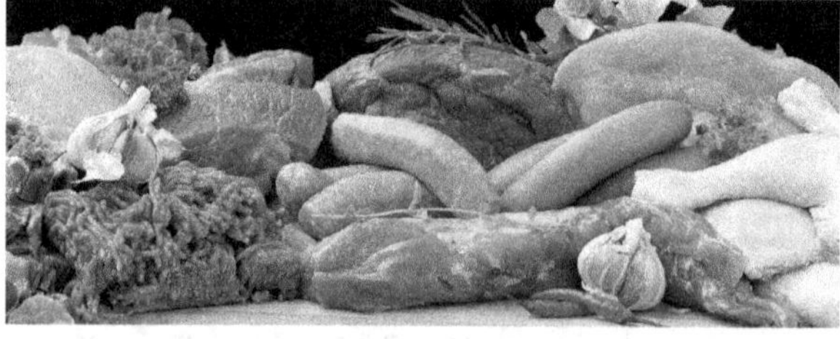

One guideline that I follow is to open any suspicious package of meat and smell it. If it smells bad, it may still be good, but I'm not going to take a chance if a meat smells peculiar.

I don't care if it is just the slime that can build up from the meat being sealed on plastic, or if it is the start of a simple mold that can be trimmed off.

Personally, I will move on to another selection or cut of meat and if it also smells bad, that's it for me with that store's meats. If this continues to happen as a particular store I will definitely change supermarkets. For more information on the world of Supermarket meats see the chapter called Meats and Supermarkets for more information on this.

One basic rule you can depend on though is; if it's on sale, then for some reason they got it cheaper than they normally do, or they have decided that is in their best interest to sell it off as soon as possible.

Is the meat old? Is the meat from a new cheaper source? Is there just too much of the particular meat in their freezer?

OK, sometimes it might be the week after the Fourth of July, or whatever, and they didn't sell as many steaks or as much hamburger than they had planned so they just want to dump it before it goes bad.

Whatever the root cause for the sale, no supermarket is going to sell a product, especially something as expensive as meats, for a lower price except that they have decided that they need to do so, and do it soon.

Traffic Management to push products

Of course you must have realized by now that the layout of a supermarket forces you to travel through the store, aisle by aisle, from the entrance to the checkout counters on a controlled path.

Think about it, you take your cart and your coupon flyer and you walk into the supermarket. The first thing you notice is that you are trapped in a series of rows that force you to walk by certain products.

This is intentionally done to make you look at and possibly put these first viewed products into your cart. These products are there for several reasons; they are either the most perishable items in the store or they are the ones with the highest profit margin.

 If you pick up; a can of red beans, a fresh baked loaf of those prominently displayed; Italian Breads, a few fresh organic tomatoes, a bag of Oranges or even a pound of sliced Ham and put it into your cart then they will have won the game.

 By selecting just a few of these items before you start looking at the other more essential items on your list then they have won the first subtle confrontation with you and your shopping budget.

At this point, you will be subtly directed up and down their aisles of canned goods, condiments, and even frozen foods.

After you have these essentials are in your cart, you will see aisles of cleaning products, kitchen tools, storage containers, and then snacks.

They want you to see and possibly buy these before you get to such items as breads, crackers, cheeses, eggs, butters and other spreads as well as milks and other dairy products.

Once they have your cart full of their preferred sales items they will force you to at least walk by their selections of beers and wines, just in case they can get yet another sale out of you.

Then there is that small area at the end of each aisle in the supermarket. This is prime display space and again, those supermarket planners are trying to get you to purchase these select items placed so conspicuously at the ends of the aisles.

If you check, these end-of-aisle items are not necessarily the best of their class or the lowest priced, but they are the ones that the supermarket chain wants to move.

In fact, often these items are displayed and priced to either clear their shelves of the item or just to draw you into that specific aisle and possibly even pick up even more of the item for your cart.

So, once you, the shopper, recognize these facts about these subtle marketing tricks that supermarkets use, you are ready to use them to your advantage.

Remember, if you pick up a can of tomato sauce that is displayed on a shelf at the entrance to the store, and later find a cheaper, and just as good, selection of the same thing on the shelf, just place the more expensive on onto the shelf and get the cheaper one.

When you do this, you will have won a small but important victory over their marketing geniuses back at their corporate headquarters.

You are there to get the best deal on the best products that you really need, and you are not there to buy a quart of mustard or ketchup that you may rarely use just because it is on sale.

Shop smart and you will save your hard earned money when you are in the supermarkets.

Supermarkets and Meats

There are basic federal standards on meats, such as; how to handle them, how they are graded, and even recommendations on when to remove them from the shelf. But there are few real and enforceable standards in place today.

Chicken and Salmonella

Salmonella is a bacterium that is the cause of the most common form of food poisoning. It is actually found on most of the Chickens sold in America.

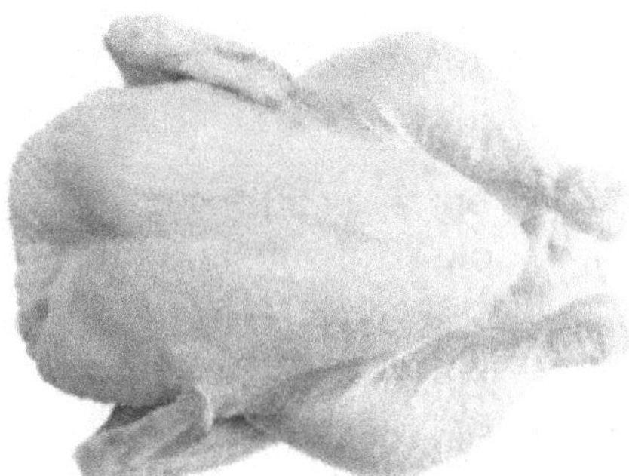

Most of the chicken on a supermarket meat shelf probably has some small level of Salmonella bacteria on it. In fact, it is the rare case if it doesn't.

The human body's digestive system and its high levels of acid will destroy most bacteria in foods, including typical levels of Salmonella.

It is recommended that you adequately cook your chicken and other fowl to the proper temperature (165F or higher, for the recommended minimum period of time. This will kill Salmonella bacteria and assure that your chicken is safe to eat.

BEEF and Sell By Dates

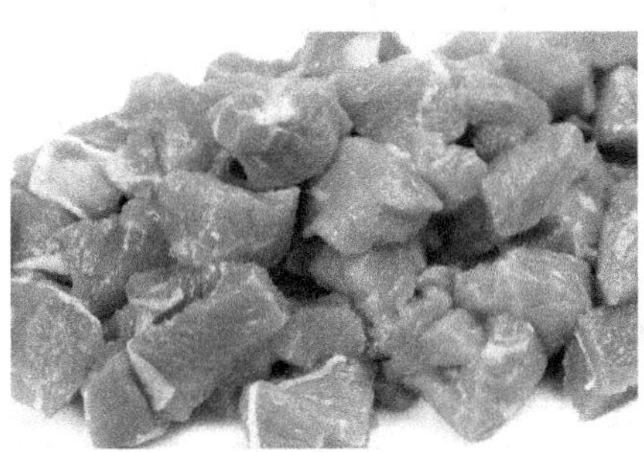

Beef, like all meats, will degrade over time and supermarkets will label them with a **Sell By Date**, which is the last day they should sell it and still allow the consumer to use it before it goes bad.

On the other hand, some beef products are preferred by customers to be properly aged before consumption.

Beef can be **Dry-Aged** which is a process that can take weeks or some beef is preferred when it is **Wet-Aged**.

See the Tip - **Aging Beef** for more on these meat-aging procedures. Remember "sell by dates" are literally just suggestions put on foods by the retail store, and not a predictable period of time set by the FDA or any other government agency.

See the chapter called **Understanding Food Freshness** for more specific recommendations on how long a period of time some foods can last beyond the "sell by date" on the label.

Some stores are very aggressive in managing their product image when it comes to meats, while others are more lenient in what they consider an acceptable shelf life.

Hamburger Storage

Packaged hamburger should be stored in a freezer if it is over three days old.

The best suggestion I can give you is to use your eyes and your nose when examining displayed meats. If it looks and smells bad, don't purchase it.

Always smell any meat you are considering purchasing, and if it smells bad then you should not purchase it.

I suggest that you **become friendly with the butcher** in your store. Be friendly, get to know him, and start asking him questions about what you pick up. They will generally give you an honest opinion of whether that particular package is OK or not, and why.

Often, older cuts of Beef, especially the ugly dried out ones, are ground up, along with some fat trimmings into Hamburger in an attempt to salvage the meat from eventually being scrapped.

And, in case you didn't know it, the "**Sell By Date**" on the old label? Well the old label is discarded and the "new" ground beef gets a brand new label, with its own "sell by date".

The black or gray color of some hamburger is normally caused by moisture and oxidation and does not indicate that the meat is bad.

By the way, **Steak Tar-Tar** or **Beef Carpaccio** is made from the Filet cut of steak. An untrimmed Filet such as what is used in these dishes, is encased in a thick layer of fat that naturally protects the meat from bacteria.

Pork Chops

Always buy fatty pork chops because the more fat you see on the chop then the better the Pork Chop will taste after it is cooked with this fat on it.

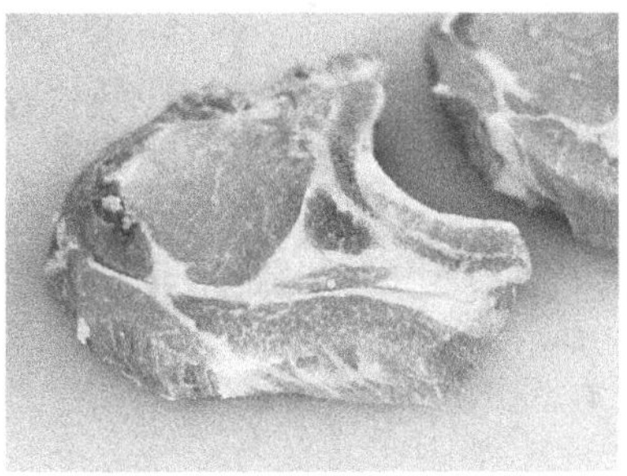

Prime Meat Grade pork chops will have a higher level of marbling in the meat and, as a result, will usually be more flavorful.

Even if you don't want to eat the fat, you should cook the chop with the fat on it and then trim away what you don't want, as you eat the juicy pork chop. You will get more of the great fat flavor with the meat and actually not be eating much fat.

Sausages

Your typical supermarket will usually have a nice variety of sausages available for their customer's selection.

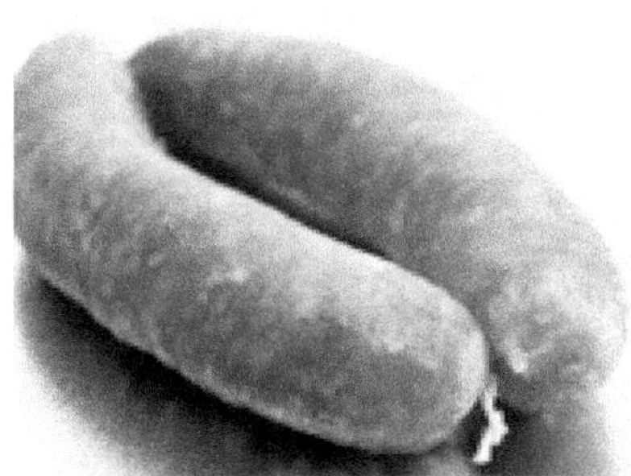

Some sausages are manufactured and delivered frozen to the retailer, while some retailers make their sausages so that they can use their excess meats and trim scraps.

Always examine the label on a manufacturers sausages, looking for the different additives that you may find listed there. Some are benign and safe while others should concern you about whether they are actually safe for you to consume.

Whenever you are buying fresh sausages, if you are not going to use them in the next couple of days, you should **always freeze them** until you do plan to use them.

GROW YOUR OWN FOODS

You don't have to own a large tract of land to grow at least some of your own foods and herbs. Many people, living in homes on very small pieces of land are able to grow a surprising number of plants, herbs and other foods.

I know of people who have only a small area on their apartment patio that are growing seasonal foods and year-round herbs for their enjoyment. Of course, the smaller the size of your land, the more inventive you must be to make the maximum use of your personal garden.

What I am saying is that anyone can have a garden of some size, if they take the time to make an annual plan and I say annual plan because, regardless of how much space you have, there are things that grow better at different times of the year.

And to be the most efficient gardener you need to have a plan that helps you plant and harvest certain seasonal foods year round by utilizing your garden space to its maximum.

How big is your Garden?

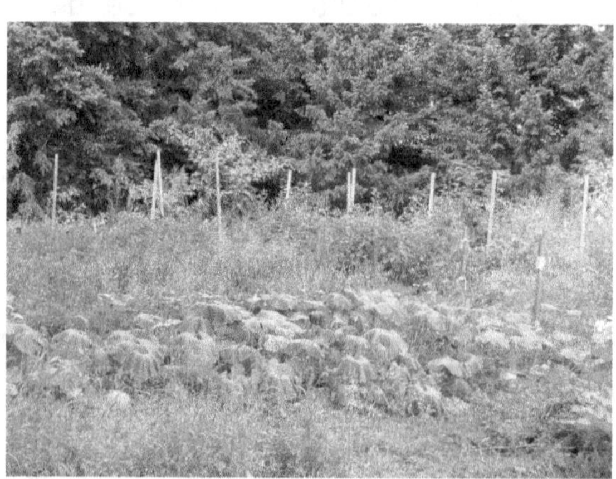

Even if you live in an apartment with very little floor space and only a few windows for light, you can grow a surprising number of vegetables and even your favorite herbs in pots.

Think about it; your own cherry tomatoes, sage, rosemary, parsley, thyme, and others of your favorite vegetables and herbs, grown in a few pots that you place strategically near your windows for the best access to sunlight.

These potted plants will grow year round and provide you with natural flavorings when you cook your favorite dishes.

And I know of people living in apartments in cities that have a small outdoor patio. Specifically, there is one lady I know of who decided that she wanted to have a functional garden more than she wanted to have a lot of pretty flowering potted plants.

The patio was not very big but it was large enough for her to build a small 8-foot by 8-foot garden. See the chapter called, How to Build a Patio Garden.

So, let's say that you do not live in an apartment but have a home, in the city and there is a small space, a very small space in fact, that you want to use for a Garden. If you have read the instructions for How to Build a Patio Garden, then you can relax a little. Building a small outside garden is much simpler. See the chapter called **How to Build a Backyard Garden.**

Of course, you can grow whatever you in your garden and you should grow what appeals to you and your tastes. But, there are certain foods that are recommended as being the best for a Survivalist when it comes to getting the most nutrition for your investment in space and labor.

See the chapter called; **Recommended Crop Foods** for a list of these important priority foods for the Survivalist gardener.

Knowing Seeds

When you get ready to plant your garden you need to know the differences in the types of plants and their seeds. By this I mean that you need to know the difference between what are called; heirloom seeds, hybrid seeds and GMO or Genetically Modified Organism Seeds.

You should remember that some plants are popular for their flavor, their hardiness, their resistance to pests and diseases and some are just popular for their productive output.

Heirloom Seeds

First of all, there are the **Heirloom seeds**. These are the seeds of plants that have been grown successfully by people for centuries and some of the seeds from each year's plantings are usually saved so they can be replanted the next year.

Many Heirloom plant seeds are so popular that they have been used continuously for 100-300 years and a few even longer. Most heirloom seeds are popular for their flavor and are typically used in family gardens and some small market gardens.

Hybrid Seeds

Hybrid Seeds are seeds collected from a hybrid plant. So, what is a hybrid plant? A hybrid plant is one that has been made from combining parts of two different plants.

For instance, many fruit trees, grape plants and others will be the result of combining the hearty root stock of one plant with the preferred fruit bearing properties of another. Many commercial plants are hybrids.

The problem with using a hybrid plant is that it will not produce the same type of seeds and unless it is a perennial like the examples above, it must be re-produced each year.

GMO Seeds

Genetically Modified Seeds are the seeds of plants that have been modified scientifically to get certain enhanced characteristics. Certain foreign characteristics are implanted into the gene of a plant, such as antibiotic resistance, along with other desired traits.

The yield of a GMO Seed is not greater than that of an unmodified plant, and only a few vegetables and plants have been approved by the FDA, such as; alfalfa, corn, cotton, tomatoes, soy, squash, and potatoes, among others.

GMO plants are preferred by commercial growers and rarely used by gardeners.

Open Pollenated Plants – There are open pollinated varieties of Heirloom plants but a few of the other varieties are also "open pollinated". Open pollenated plants will grow each year and the gathered seeds, when replanted will produce the same variety, year after year.

Organic Certified Seeds

Organic plants are produced under very strict standards and seeds from plants that are labeled as "Organic" are not necessarily heirloom, but are certified to have been grown under these strict Federal standards.

HERBS and FOODS you can GROW INDOORS

The Survivalist can start small in their quest for more control of their life and lifestyle. One way is for them to grow certain of their Herbs and some plants indoors.

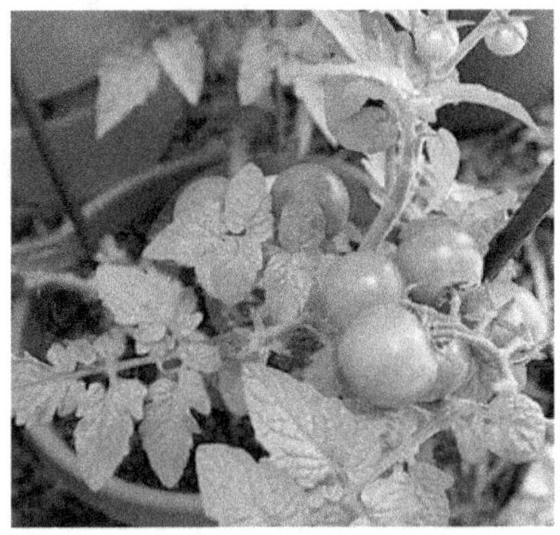

Whether in an apartment or a home, there is always room for a few well-placed pots that can contain nutritious and healthy food items.

Doing this is not only a good way to save money it also gives you small amounts of these foods year-round.

To be successful growing foods indoors you only need a few items and you are on your way to a better lifestyle. Go to a few of your local Garden supply stores and talk to one of their gardening "experts".

Unless you are looking to grow something exotic, they will tell you that you need the following to **get started**:
1. A Terra Cotta pot and water plate to set it on. I recommend a 1-2 gallon pot depending on the expected size of the plant.
2. A watertight plastic or metal tray to set the pots on to avoid spills and stains.
3. A bag of gravel or rocks. The rocks should be around 1-inch in diameter.
4. One or more bags of potting soil depending on how many plants you are going to start.
5. Grow lights if your plants cannot be kept near a window with access to sunlight.
6. A small bag of fertilizer, Organic or a Natural Fertilizer if not Organic.
7. A selection of your favorite herbs or food plants to grow. Get the advice of your local "expert" on planting them properly.

Once you have collected your materials and are at home, use your supplies to **prepare your new food growing pots** as follows:
1. Fill the pots to about 1/3 full with the rocks.
2. Cover the layer of rocks with the Potting Soil up to about 1-inch of the top of the pot.

3. Mix in a small amount of the fertilizer (about 1-tbs. for a gallon pot) into the potting soil and then pack the soil down.
4. Wet the soil with water and, after a half-hour or so, press it down again.
5. Make a hole in the soil and insert roots of the plant up to the main stem, or insert the seeds about 1-inch deep in the soil.
6. Cover the seeds with the surrounding dirt or press the surrounding dirt firmly around the plant.
7. Cover the dirt with a little more loose potting soil and water the plant thoroughly.
8. Place the pot near the window or under the grow light and wait to enjoy your homegrown treats.
    NOTE: Be sure to know how much and how often to water your plants. Too much water can be just as bad for a plant as too little. Typically, you should water most Herbs every two weeks.

Recommended Indoor Herbs

Here are some recommended Herbs for you to plant an indoor garden. They should adapt well to an indoor environment and produce useful Herbs for you year round; **Basil, Bay Leaf, Cilantro, Chervil, Chive, Lavender, Oregano, Parsley, Rosemary, Sage, Tarragon** and **Thyme** to name just some of the more popular.

Again, you can grow your own fresh Herbs and have better tasting dishes to serve your family and friends when you use them and you will also enjoy their fresh fragrances in your house.

Try using the leaves of such plants as lavender, lemon balm and other fragrant herbs in a potpourri to give the air in your home a fresh natural scent, and you will also find that still others go well in herbal teas.

How to Build a Patio Garden

Anyone can build a small patio garden regardless of whether they only have a small piece of open land on their property at the rear or side their house or even if they only have a patio space attached to their apartment in a city.

There are many people whose home does not have an actual yard, but some do have a Patio that could be used for growing at least some of their favorite fresh foods.

A Patio garden is actually relatively simple to build and maintain, but it will take a little planning and perseverance to get one started.

Water Drainage Control

The only real and very important difference when planning one is that with a Patio garden is you need to find a way to manage your water runoff from your garden area.

Most apartments with patios already have some type of water runoff management that will have been built into the building's design.

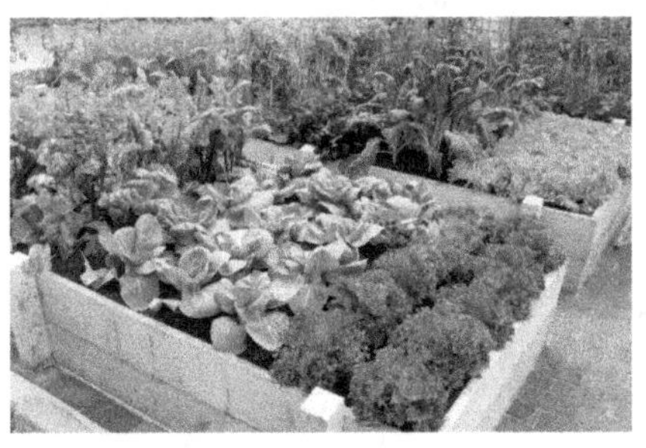

You still don't want to irritate your neighbors living below you with your excess garden water washing dirt and other garden debris down and onto their patio at peak rain periods.

So, in order to "keep the peace" so to speak, some water management must be included into your design work. Your Patio garden can be pretty much any size, but for simplicity's sake, I will describe the design of an 8-foot by 8-foot garden space for a Patio.

Patio Garden Construction

You should start with the base for the small Patio Garden and use one or more pieces of outdoor plywood placed on top of some cheap cinder bricks that will elevate your garden above the floor of the patio itself.

Both of these can be purchased at your local home repair and garden center. Most of these stores will also cut your plywood to your desired dimensions for free.

Donald W Bobbitt

The reason I picked an 8x8-foot square design was that you would typically find that sheets of plywood are sold in 4x8-foot sections in the US and picking these dimensions simplifies your construction and overall costs by using standard sized materials.

Space the Cinder Bricks every two feet and then position your plywood over the bricks. With this spacing you can get away with using a 3/8-inch thick sheet of plywood for your garden base.

Please note that you can get these 4x8 sheets cut in half for easier handling if you are going to transport the plywood to your house yourself.

Transporting such large items can be made easier if you have a friend with a pickup truck or open van who will help you. Bribe them with promises of fresh vegetables when your first crop comes in.

Retaining Wall

Once your plywood is firmly positioned, build a wall around the edges at least 10-inches high using cheap landscaping blocks that you can again find in the garden section of your local Home Center. If you think these might be too heavy for your patio, try having some plywood cut in lengths that are only 12-inches wide.

These blocks come in many specific sizes so if you know the overall size of the desired walls, in this case 8x8, it only takes a few calculations to select the right ones for your dirt retaining wall.

Let's say they have 6-inch wide by 6-inch high stackable blocks in different lengths. You can get seven 12-inch long blocks and one six-inch long block for each side of your retaining wall and they will go together perfectly.

 Then you can place another layer on top of the first and you will have a 12-inch high retaining wall built onto your plywood base.

This calculates to a total of 7x4x2 or 56 of the 12-inch landscaping blocks and 4x2 or 8 of the six-inch blocks to finish your basic patio garden structure.

More simply, the 12-inch plywood lengths can be nailed together and to the base plywood for a nice border, if you have basic carpenter skills.

Water Liner

Now, at this point you can just throw dirt into the garden bed but I would suggest that you enhance it with a few features.

First, I would get a sturdy plastic tarp and line the garden bed with it making sure that the tarp is large enough to reach the top inside edges of the landscaping blocks (or plywood).

By using a cheap glue on the plywood and on the inside of the blocks before putting the tarp in place it will be bonded to the garden bottom and walls and this will help keep the tarp in place and even give a little support to the walls.

Drainage Bed

Secondly, if you want a way to keep your soil moist but also avoid having problems with mold and even root-rot, I suggest that you put a cheap drain field on top of the tarp.

The simplest drain field would be one like what describe below.

I suggest that you purchase several pieces of plastic water pipe, at least ½-inch inside diameter. Glue them together using the same type of plastic plumbing elbows giving you good coverage for draining the whole garden area.

Using a small drill bit, around 1/8-inch or so, drill a row of holes into the pipe, spaced about 6-inches apart and on opposite sides of the pipe.

Remove one of the shorter landscape blocks from the lower wall, cut a small hole in the water liner and insert the drain end of the plastic pipe assembly into your garden and to the center of the garden space.

It should be protruding about 4-6-inches from the wall, then seal around the pipe with a silicone sealant. Fill the rest of the opening where the landscaping block was removed with a modified block or a piece of wood or whatever you can find that will support the upper layer and the plastic liner adequately.

Then place a bed of drainage rocks over the pipe. This can be achieved by placing about a two to three inch layer of landscape rock onto the bottom tarp and drainage pipe.

If you are worrying about the weight of the rock on your patio, you can even use Lava Rock that is very lightweight relative to other landscaping rocks.

Drainage Bed Shield

I suggest that you use a drainage shield over the layer of rocks. Again, at your Home and Garden Center, get a large enough piece of what is called landscaping paper and cover all of the rocks. This material will impede the growth of your gardens plant roots through and into rock and eventually impeding the drainage of excess water from your garden.

Planting Soil

You can now fill your patio garden with about 6-inches of good planting soil or other recommended soil. You can purchase bags of simple topsoil and spread it over the drainage shield or you can pick one of the more expensive but usually very good soil mixtures that already have fertilizers included.

Whatever you pick, you will need to water it down and allow the soil to settle a couple of times before you plant anything. Often, six inches of loose soil can pack down to just 2-3inches of usable soil, so be prepared to add soil after the original layer has packed.

Ready to Use Patio Garden

This patio garden is a simple design that you can build on and improve, as you see fit, over time. But regardless, at this point, you have a great place, on your patio that you can use for planting your favorite fresh vegetables, herbs and other plants.

Additionally, with just a little planning you can get multiple "plantings" over the same year in your patio garden.

Build a simple VERTICAL GARDEN

Imagine having your own pyramid of food, just outside your door.

There are so many ways to grow more of your own favorite foods in a relatively small space, but I think you would like this idea the best.

If you do have an outside area that is anywhere up to the size of 8-feet by 10-feet, with good access to the Sun and rain, then a vertical garden can provide you with a lot of food in a very small space.

The construction is actually easy if you can picture placing two wooden pallets together in a triangle formation.

First of all calculate the size of wooden frames needed to fit in your potential garden area where you can grow foods and still walk around the assembly. Using these dimensions, go to your local garden store or building supply store and have them calculate the materials you need.

Build two wooden frames out of 2x4 boards with several boards spaced parallel and 12-18 inches apart on the frames. Attach the two frames together with a couple of door hinges. Stand the two joined frames upright and spread the bottoms apart to a gap of about 1/3 of the height, giving you a nice open triangle framework.

Brace the bottoms of the frames to the ground with stakes to avoid them slipping apart from the weight you will be adding as you build your garden.

Hanging Pots: Purchase some cheap plastic flowerpots that can hold about a gallon of dirt each. Drill three holes in the edge of the pots and attach three wires to the holes and together about 10-inches above the pot. Mount a hook to the twisted together three wires attached to the tops edges of the pots and fill the pots with dirt.

Add some cheap **screw-in hooks** onto the inside of the now horizontal boards on the frames about 12-18 inches apart. These will be used to hang your old planting pots.

Hang the pots onto the frame hooks and plant your favorite vegetables in these pots. Water them regularly, and you will soon have an amazing crop of fresh foods growing in those pots for your enjoyment.

You can even **plant vine vegetables** such as cucumbers in pots sitting on the ground at the base of the frame and run the growing vines up the frame. When the cucumbers are grown, they will be hanging over your head ready for picking.

Just imagine, **Potatoes, Carrots, Onions and such growing at your feet while Tomatoes, Squash, Peas, Green Beans, Peppers, Cucumbers, your favorite Herbs** and even **small Melons** are growing over your head, and all in the area of your little vertical garden.

How to Build a Backyard Garden

Let's assume that you have a really large backyard, with anywhere

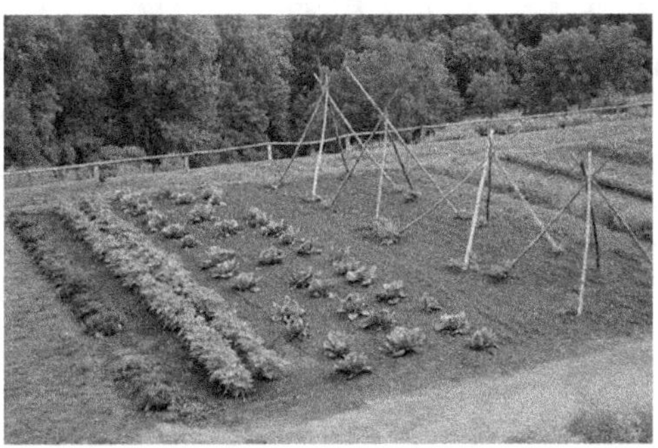

from as little as 200 square feet to as much as 2000 square feet that you want to use for your garden.

There are a few things that I can tell you that will help you build a garden that produces abundant crops of your favorite foods and herbs, efficiently and with minimal problems.

And yes, I said crops.

Once you get to this size of garden space available, you will be able to grow enough of your favorite foods to not only feed yourself and your family but also be able to can, freeze and store some for later use.

Pick Your Site

Your garden site should be located where it will get a good portion of the day's direct sunlight. Adequate sunlight is necessary for any garden vegetable to grow and flourish.

Along with adequate sunlight, your garden will need to get plenty of fresh air. Good air flow will not only allow for good pollination but it will also help avoid problems with molds and certain bacteria.

Sloped land makes a Better Garden

Try to plant your garden on land that has at least a little slope to it. A flat garden will not drain adequately and excess water in the soil can not only harm your crop but also provide a breeding ground for numerous harmful bacteria.

And, if your garden spot is sloped, plant your crops in rows that go across the slope, rather than up and down. Doing this will contain the rains waters and allow the water time to seep into the ground rather than run away too quickly.

Donald W Bobbitt

Preparing the Soil

Your garden soil will need to be prepared properly. I recommend that if you can grab a handful of your soil easily and crush it into a ball that then breaks up easily, your soil will at least absorb water easily.

If it also smells slightly musty and you can actually find worms and bugs living in it, then it is probably a healthy soil.

But, if you want to have a good garden, I recommend that you take a sample to your County Farm Agent and ask them to test the soil for you. They can give you a detailed analysis of your soil including which nutrients that it might need added for you to grow good crops.

These agencies often do this testing for free or at least at a low cost. Another option might be for you to purchase your own soil testing kit at your local garden shop.

Soil pH Levels:

One key thing to know about your soil is its pH level. The pH level is essentially a measure of the amount of lime in your soil.

A pH level of less than 7.0 means your soil is acidic which is typical of wet climates, while one higher than 7.0 is considered Alkaline and is typical of Dry climates.

The pH level of your soil is important because different vegetables prefer different pH levels to grow well and produce larger crop yields.

Selecting the Best Crops

As I have already mentioned, your garden is yours and you should plant and grow what suits you and your tastes.

At the same time, there are certain foods that are recommended for Survivalists because they are; hearty plants, easily grown and produce highly nutritious crops in relatively large quantities.

See the chapter called; Recommended Crop Foods for a list of these recommended foods.

Using Planting Dates and Maturity periods

Plants have different; planting dates, soil temperature requirements for gestation and periods of time it takes for them to mature.

Knowing these can give you an advantage when you select and eventually plant your crops.

See the attached table labeled: **Table-B1-1 Planting Times for Common Foods** to see a useful list for many popular foods.

Managing Weeds

Weeds will show up in every garden. It's just a fact of life. So many weeds have small seeds that blow around with the winds and can land in anyone's garden.

Weeds love all of the things that you have provided for your garden foods; good soil, plenty of water and great fertilizers.

So it should be no surprise that once they take root, they thrive. A good gardener though should have no problem managing weeds. It just takes a strong back, a good hoe and a little time to control weeds.

The process is simple, find a weed, chop down and below its roots, a twist of the wrist to turn the roots up and you are done.

Then flip the weed plant to an open area between the garden rows, and fill the spot where the weed was with some loose soil using the same hoe.

With the weeds roots sticking up in the air, and no longer in the soil the weed plant will wither up, almost before your eyes. Later, rake the weeds up and pile them in your compost pile to salvage their nutrients.

Mulch: Many people will use mulch to control weeds in their garden. Usually mulch is made from such things as rotting wood chips, wood bark and other such materials.

Landscape cloth: Commercial growers will often shape their planting rows, and cover them with sheets of garden landscape paper to block weeds and simple cut a small hole in the paper where they plant a pre-grown seedling.

Old Newspapers: I have friends who take this yet another step for their small garden and once the plants come up, they will spread old newspapers around the plant control weeds. One advantage of newspapers is that they will eventually rot so they can be plowed up with the garden at the end of the growing season.

Harvesting your Crops

Determining when a fruit or plant is ready for harvesting is a learned thing. With some foods, the determining factor is going to be a combination of the color, smell or firmness of the fruit. You just have to use your senses and over time you will get good at this.

So, let's say your crop is ready to harvest. Each food, fruit or plant can be pulled or cut from the plant differently. For instance an Apple or an Orange will easily release from the limb if it is ripe. So, just a light tug should be all that is needed.

A tomato, on the other hand, will ripen and still not release from the plant easily. They will require a firm tug to pull the fruit free. Of course, a tomato's color tells you that the fruit is ripe and ready.

Always wear gloves when harvesting your crop because even the safest fertilizers and pesticides can be harsh to your skin.

Washing the food

Right after harvesting your crop you should always give the individual fruits or vegetables a good washing to remove as much as possible of any residual chemicals that might be on the crops surface.

Take extra care to clean certain areas of the crop. The flowering end and the stem area will collect more of any sprayed chemicals.

Leaf vegetables will have higher concentrations not only on the leaves, but also at the junction of the leaves, near the root area. Also, the root area of such foods as Celery, Beets, Potatoes and Carrots should get the same special attention.

Storing your Crops

When crops come in, you are probably going to be stunned by how much food you have to contend with, and a lot of it at one time.

So, you can either be the guy handing out free homegrown food to their friends, or you can be the guy who prepared ahead of time. Here are some things you can do so that you get the most from your garden.

Canning Foods

If you have the materials and storage space you should Can your excess fresh grown foods. Properly canned foods can last for several years stored on a shelf in a cool dry place in your homes pantry, or basement.

Green Beans, Lima Beans, Squash, Tomatoes, Cucumbers and other such foods are great foods that can be canned or even pickled. In fact Corn, once you remove the kernels from the husk, also cans well.

Crop Shelf Storage

Some foods such as potatoes and tomatoes can be stored fresh for weeks. Pick a cool dry place and place newspapers onto the shelves then lay the potatoes or tomatoes loosely onto the paper.

The tomatoes, especially the green ones will keep for weeks and the Potatoes can keep for months.

So, always watch for the last days before the coming first winter's frost, and pull those green tomatoes and store them on paper lined shelves so that you will get to eat them for several more weeks.

Hot Peppers also keep well stored on shelves but do even better if you string them together and hang them to dry for later use.

Dried Foods – Many plants, and especially herbs and spices lend themselves well to drying. Drying plants and seeds is a relatively simple process.

The cleaned plants must be laid out in a sunny area with a low humidity.

On a small scale there are kits/tools that you can use to dry some foods. On a larger scale, the concept is the same but the tools needed may be a little more complicated.

Managing the Debris

One thing that you are going to realize as you use your garden is that there is going to be a lot of debris to get rid of at certain times during the year. Some of this debris will be made of plastics and other materials that are not biodegradable.

Non-Biodegradable Debris - These items need to be handled and disposed of properly. Here are a few tips to reduce your work and allow you to manage them efficiently.

For a small garden just place a large garbage can near the garden and as you use bagged or packaged products just place all of the plastic bags and such into the trashcan.

Donald W Bobbitt

Do your part for the environment by taking the larger quantities of plastic and metal debris to a Recycle Center so that it can be used again after it is processed.

Biodegradable Debris - Then there are the biodegradable items. With these items, you can also use trashcans or you can start a dry pile near your garden,

A dry pile is just a place that you pile your trimmed portions of plants or bushes and wait for them to dry out. Once dry, this debris is much lighter and easier to handle.

Or, you can take this opportunity to build and construct a good old-fashioned Compost Pit and get wonderful reusable fodder to fertilize you next year's garden. See the chapter on Building a Compost Pit.

Allow the Soil to Rest

Farmers know that using a plot of land whether it is a small truck garden or one that takes up several acres, over and over for the same crops will eventually rob the soil of valuable nutrients.

This goes for your home garden also. Ideally, you should rotate the crops grown on a piece of land regularly.

Some farmers will plant their soil land a re-invigorating crop, such as Soy or Peas, every 3-4 years and when the crop is grown, they just turn the mature plants back into the soil and allow the soil to rest for a season and absorb the nutrient rich plants.

But there are other alternatives available for the small gardener.
* You can add bags of soil to your garden and till this fresh soil into your garden.
* You can take soil samples to your county agent and have your soil tested to find out what fertilizers and nutrients need replenishing.
* And, depending on the size of your desired garden, and the amount of open land you have, just move your garden to another spot for a few years.

Recommended Crop Foods

Growing a garden is a personal thing and as such, you need to select crops that suit your personal tastes. For instance, I mention Beets below. Some people love Beets, even whole nations consume Beets in large quantities.

I, on the other hand, detest beets, regardless of the way you cook or spice them up, and you will not find me planting these in my garden.

Anyway, the foods listed below are highly recommended as crops for the Retro-Survivalist. They are typically very hearty plants that provide valuable nutrients when consumed.

There are so many great foods that you can plant in your garden but these are recommended as the best options for garden planting by a number of gardening experts who specialize in providing information for growing healthy foods.

BEETS

Beets, as with Turnips are a gardeners essential. The roots can be stored for later use during the winter and the greens are not only nutritious but also very tasty when cooked properly.

BROCCOLI

Broccoli is actually a member of the cabbage family and is a highly nutritious food that is relatively easy to grow. It likes sandy soil and lots of sunshine but prefers cool climates so it is typically grown as a Spring or Fall crop.

Broccoli Leaves

Although we usually discard them, one ounce of Broccoli leaves can provide 90% of the daily requirement for Vitamin A where the popular floret will provide only 3%. Cook the leaves as you would Spinach or eat them raw in a salad.

COLLARDS

Collards are also a member of the cabbage family and the leaves provide nutrient rich greens throughout the Summer. They are easy to grow and have always been the most popular in the southern parts of the US.

CORN

Field Corn is a plant that you should have in your garden. Some varieties and even hybrids will have a sweet flavor and are great for immediate consumption. Regular field corn though, is not as sweet tasting as some other varieties, but it is best for drying and then grinding into cornmeal.

When compared with wheat, corn is a more productive crop for the same size piece of land.

GARLIC, ONIONS and LEEKS

Garlic, Onions and Leeks are fantastic plants that are easy to plant and care for. They are not only nutritious and loaded with their own unique flavor, but they also have important medicinal applications.

Although they do take a while to grow, you can start them inside and then re-plant the seedlings after the final spring frost is over if you want your crop to mature earlier.

GREEN BEANS

Green Beans are so nutritious and flavorful that almost everyone with a garden wants to grow them. The Pole-Bean variants will give you the most production than others, so stick to these varieties.

And there are varieties that are great for drying for later use, called dry-soup beans.

Green Beans are often consumed fresh, but some people will freeze them or even can some of their crop for later use. They are not only easy to grow, but they are hardy plants requiring very little care.

HAZEL NUTS (Filberts)

The Hazel Nut, or Filbert Nut, is a hearty nut whose kernel provides essential nutrients and grows on a small tree. A newly planted tree will bear fruit in 3-4 years. Although the nuts are small, they are easy to remove from the shell and store well.

KALE

Kale is not as popular as Collard for fresh and tasty greens and the plant is not quite as productive, but the nutritional value is just as good and the flavor is preferred by many people, particularly that of the Russian Red Kale. White Kale is heartier and can thrive in hotter temperatures.

OKRA

Okra is a vegetable that is grown and eaten primarily in the southern parts of the US, but the plant itself is hearty and easy to grow. An Okra plant is highly productive and it can be frozen, generally without blanching, for later use. Okra is popular when breaded and fried and is often used in Gumbos and other Cajun dishes.

PARSLEY

Parsley is a hearty plant that does not take up a lot of garden space and can even be grown indoors in pots for year-round use. Parsley provides high levels of Vitamin-C and A as well as containing a high mineral content.

PARSNIPS

Before potatoes were introduced into Europe the Parsnip was the main starchy root vegetable grown.

The parsnip is easy to grow and cultivate and they can be left in the ground and pulled as needed throughout the winter (if the ground isn't frozen).

It is as nutritious root that provides high levels of calories and carbohydrates.

PEANUTS

The Peanut plant is prolific in that one plant will produce surprising large quantities of peanuts in the right soil.

The peanut is a high protein food that although being high in fat is relatively low in Carbohydrates.

PEPPERS, HOT

There are hundreds of Hot Peppers available for you to grow, and once you do grow a couple of varieties for yourself, you will always have some in your garden. Hot Peppers store well whether they are just bagged and frozen, or if they are strung and hung in a dry area of your home.

Take care when actually coking with Hot Peppers because peppers from the same plant can give a wide variety in their "hotness".

Here are a few of my favorite varieties:

Banana Peppers

Banana Peppers are great fresh or if they are canned. They have a slightly spicy flavor as compared with others and are great on sandwiches and in salads. They can be caned or pickled easily with the addition of a few spices.

Cayenne Peppers

A couple of Cayenne Pepper plants can provide the average gardener with an adequate quantity of these hot treats for the whole year. Pick them as they ripen and turn red and start using them in your favorite spicy dishes.

Jalapeno Peppers

JALAPENO Peppers are a favorite pepper for many people in many nations. They provide a nice kick to any dish, especially if you use the seeds and interior ribs for cooking, as they are usually the hottest parts of the pepper itself.

POTATOES

If you have a variety of Potato plant that is acclimated to your local environment, and weather conditions and if you grow them in good soil then the plants will provide you with large crops.

Potatoes are nutritious and are high in Calories, Proteins and Minerals. They can be stored for months in a cool, dark and dry place.

SOYBEANS

Soybean plants are a protein-rich crop that produces abundant amounts of the vegetable. They are a versatile food because they are used to make Tofu, Soy Milk and Tempeh among others and are great consumed as baked nuts, and sprouts.

They are very nutritious and easy to grow.

SUMMER SQUASH

There are literally hundreds of varieties of Squash available to the gardener, but the most popular are Zucchini Squash and Yellow Squash.

Zucchini Squash grows on a vine and can grow to large sizes up to 2-feet long. It is better to harvest the smaller ones as they will be much more tender than the larger ones and they will also have lass seeds in them.

Yellow Squash is also a popular plant of the gourd family that grows to a nice size but it is best if it is harvested when smaller. Its bright color and mild flavor make it a favorite in cooked dishes as well as in fresh salads.

Both of these popular types of Squash are easily grown, harvested and they cook well, and there are thousands of recipes available for using them to make breads, entrees, salads, casseroles, etc. They can even be frozen, canned or pickle.

SUNFLOWER SEEDS

The Sunflower plant is a hardy one that you can grow on the periphery of your garden or along a fence line.

They will produce seeds that can either be dried for later use or the plants themselves can be planted until they sprout. Once they sprout, pull them from the ground, remove the shell and eat the young sprouts.

The seeds themselves can be dried and stored for later consumption.

SWEET POTATOES

Sweet Potatoes can be a productive crop if planted and tended properly. They are high in Carotene, Iron and Vitamin-B, and they can be stored for an extended time into the winter.

Even the leaves are high in these same nutrients and can be added to fresh salad greens for a nice change in flavor.

TOMATOES

Tomatoes are one vegetable that nearly everyone agrees should be planted in your garden. If planted and tended properly these hearty fruits of the tomato plant can be canned, dried and frozen with ease.

There are literally hundreds of varieties of tomato plants for you to choose from and most people migrate towards the Heirloom varieties or at least the more hearty, productive and disease resistant varieties to plant.

If you decide that you want to save seeds for future cultivation, be sure to use open-pollinated tomato varieties to assure that you get good hearty plants and healthy fruits next year from the seeds.

TURNIPS

Turnips are known to have been grown for food as far back as 2000 BC. They are highly nutritious and you can eat every part of the plant.

The **Roots** can be stored for the winter and the stalks, also known as Raab, are a favorite dish for many people in the Fall season.

The **Greens** are the part of the plant that is the highest in nutritional value, and they taste delicious when cooked properly.

WHEAT

Even though it is generally considered a food that is grown in massive quantities, many experts recommend that even the small gardener can grow a useable amount of Wheat if they plan their garden properly.

Wheat can be grown to the sprout level and then the sprouts can be ground into dough for baking or it can be grown to the grass stage of development and "juiced" to gather the rich nutrients it contains.

And the seeds of the mature plant can, of course be ground into wheat flour for use in making bread dough.

OK, OK! There are a lot of other common vegetables that you can grow in your garden. This is especially true as you travel to different regions with widely different temperatures, altitudes, soils, and access to water.

But, start with these popular options and customize your selections over time to suit your location, growing skills and personal tastes. And, if you want to get your crop to mature as soon as possible, you need to know when to plant each vegetable, and you can check out table **B1-1 Planting Times for Foods** for a good reference.

Understanding FERTILIZERS and Pest Control

What are Fertilizers?

In addition to requiring the right environment to thrive, all food plants require certain nutrients and, at times, special chemicals in order to grow properly.

In a truly natural, forest or field or mountainside you will find many plants growing that have adapted to the specific light, water, seasonal and soil conditions that exist in that area. These plants have adapted to their environment over centuries and are able to thrive and reproduce there.

But when you grow a garden you will find that you have two serious problems. Most garden vegetables grown today have been bred to produce a proper crop under far more specialized conditions than nature typically provides, in the wild. For example, a tomato plant growing in the wild might have only a few tomatoes on it while one grown in a garden is expected to generate a dozen or even more tomatoes on it.

Many garden plants have been bred to product large and abundant crops only if planted properly, in the right amount of sunlight, given specific amounts of water and drainage, and acceptable amounts of the right nutrients.

To this end, you need to understand what fertilizers are and how to decode their strange names and applications.

There are essentially three levels of required nutrients needed for most plants to grow. The first necessary level of nutrients includes the elements normally taken by the plant from the air, and these are Carbon, Hydrogen and Oxygen.

The second level of required nutrients are required in different levels by different plants and they are Nitrogen, Phosphorous, and Potassium (or Potash).

 A bag of fertilizer will usually have three numbers labeled on the bag, such as 10-8-12. This means that the specific fertilizer mixture contains; 10% Nitrogen, 8% Phosphorous and 12% Potassium. The rest of the bags content is often just filler and is useless to the plants.

Donald W Bobbitt

The third level of often-required nutrients, called micronutrients is Calcium, Magnesium and Sulfur. Along with these are some other specialized nutrients that many plants can need including Boron, Cobalt, Copper, Iron, Manganese, Molybdenum and Zinc. All of these necessary chemicals are typically available in healthy soil.

To fertilize and encourage a plants growth, under most conditions, only the standard three chemicals; Nitrogen, Phosphorous and Potassium, are needed to give a food plant what it needs.

The typical bag of fertilizer will contain instructions for how much should be spread onto the soil for proper plant growth.

ORGANIC Fertilizers

There are a number of special Organic fertilizers available in garden shops for use by the interested grower.

Some of the more widely used organic fertilizers are; **Blood Meal, Compost, Composted Manure, Cottonseed Meal, Fish Emulsion, Green Sand** and **Super Phosphate** among others. A gardener can easily check on these on the web, if they want to grow more naturally fed foods.

PESTICIDES

The bane of every gardener is the existence of pest insects that will pounce invariably onto your beautiful crops and eat them before your very eyes.

Although certain insects are necessary and desired because they aid in the cross-pollination of many crop plants, most are just pests that need to be managed.

Do not use dangerous Pesticide Chemicals

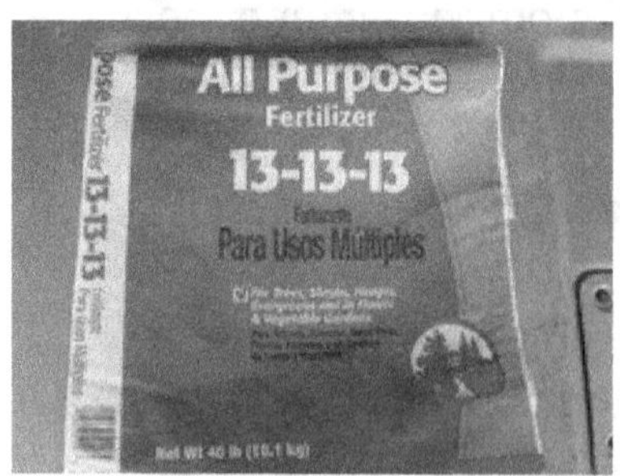

A responsible gardener will not use most of the garden chemicals that are on the market today.

Many have already been proven to be unhealthy on one form or another and many more are being found to be just as dangerous for human consumption almost every day.

Alternative methods of pest control, especially for the gardener, are typically cheaper to use than these chemicals that are available at every garden supply.

Chemical Pesticide Dangers

To control insects, there are many types of pesticides available. Your typical pesticide is a chemical concoction or biological mixture that either kills or incapacitates the pest.

They are classified as; herbicides, insecticides, fungicides, to name a few that are pest specific.

The problem with most pesticides is that they can also have an effect on the health of a human who might come in contact with them, thus making many of them toxic to one degree or another.

"Not so Bad" Chemicals.

So, now that I've banned the use of all chemicals, at least in your mind, I have to qualify my statements against all chemicals.

In all honesty, there are some effective chemicals that are simple and safe to use on garden foods and plants if they are used properly. Remember to read those labels and look up the definitions as well as the good and the bad points on their use, before you turn to chemical pest controls.

Hydrogen Peroxide as a Pest Control

I will mention one chemical that can do a good job controlling insects and that is Hydrogen Peroxide. Mix a solution of 3% Hydrogen Peroxide and Distilled water in a sprayer. Then just spray the leaves of your infected food plant and the insects will slowly die.

The Hydrogen will be absorbed into the insect's shells and kill them. And, the Hydrogen Peroxide itself will slowly break down into its base elements of Hydrogen and Oxygen, leaving no polluting chemical residue.

Alternative Pest Control Methods

There are even some popular types of pest control machines and devices that can be used to effectively and safely to control pests without harming Humans.

Some of the more popular non-Toxic pest control tools are:

Ultraviolet lights, Sound Generators, Insect Traps, Ground Vibrators, Water Treatment units, and **Air Treatment units** to name a few of the most popular.

Each of these has been shown to provide some level of pest control that is effective and at the same time not dangerous to human health.

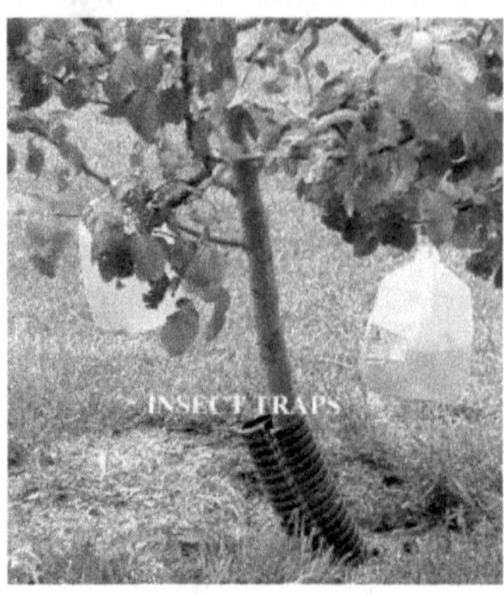

Many farmers have found that there are often even more natural ways to control specific pests quite efficiently.

See the chapter; Natural Insect Repellants for information on plants that will repel certain insects.

By applying a more natural attack strategy against your garden pests you will find that your garden produces safer and healthier produce for you and your family.

Natural and Other Insect Repellants

Probably the most popular insect repellant used today is the one called **DEET**, for short. It is a chemical combination that was first used during the Vietnam War as a strong mosquito repellant, for the prevention of malaria in the troops.

Once it is sprayed, it works for up to twelve hours before it breaks down into harmless components. But, this spray itself is toxic, if not used properly.

There are other methods used to control certain insects that do not call for using toxic chemicals, more natural ways.

PLANTS INSECTS HATE

There are some plants that, if planted strategically, will keep some insects away.

Add certain plants to your garden that will draw the good insects and they can help keep your predator Insect population down.

Flowering plants such as **Daisies**, **Mints**, **Rosemary** and **Sunflowers**, to name a few are great natural Insect repellants.

Planting a few of these strategically around your garden will work great for most gardens. Here are some of these GOOD plants and what you can use them for, in your garden or even in flowerpots in your home

BASIL

Besides being a popular and tasty herb used extensively for flavoring foods, Basil is not liked by some insects.

In fact, the essential oil extracted from Basil can be used in a spray bottle to repel Mosquitos.

CATNIP

Everyone knows that the catnip plant is useful for "relaxing" the family pet cat. The plant is a perennial that has a nice and soothing, minty aroma and you will often find that many cat owners will have a flowerpot somewhere in their house with a catnip plant in it.

You can dry the leaves of the Catnip plant and sew them into a simple cloth bag that your cat will enjoy playing with for days.

The Catnip plant contains a chemical (**Nepetalactone**) that, when purchased in Essential Oil form (the process for making the oil is relatively complex), is useful as a natural repellant for other insects such as: **Cockroaches, Flies, Mosquitos** and even **Termites.**

DAISIES

Grow Daisy plants to draw certain pest insects away from your garden. The blooms of Daisies draw such pest insects as; **Cutworms, Longhorn Beetle, Sunflower Moth, Midge, Thistle Caterpillar** and **Wire Worms** to name just a few.

GARLIC

The strong flavor and odor emitted by Garlic cloves make them repellant not only to animals and birds but also for insects. There is an extract made from Garlic that is used in some places as an insect repellant, if you do not mind the smell yourself.

Try planting some garlic in a flower pot or hanging some garlic on a string on your porch to reduce the insects near you.

GERANIUM

The flowers of the Geranium plant or specifically the **Rose Geranium** is known to repel insects due to the compound inside the plant called *geraniol*.

But, they also draw other insects; specifically honey bees, to them.

The Geranium is a good plant for cleaning the air, and medically it is used to improve glucose levels and help with digestion.

LAVENDER

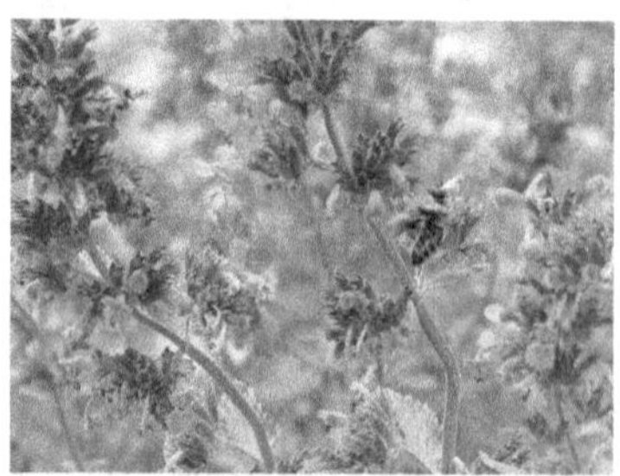

Lavender is a plant that grows cultivated as well as in the wild across the USA.

The blooms are a bright purple and it is a popular landscape plant as well as being used as a herbal treatment for insect bites and stings.

Simply blend dried Lavender flowers with Olive Oil and use it to sooth insect bites.

LEMONGRASS

The essential oil made from Lemongrass makes a great insect repellant overall, but take care because while it repels some insects, it **also draws bees.**

It is a great plant to have around the perimeter of your garden because the extra pollination by the bees will give you great fruit and vegetable yields.

MARIGOLD

The tagetes species of Marigolds, not the calendulas species has strong insect repellant properties. The blooms will not only repel mosquitoes but there are numerous other pest insects that Marigolds will repel will from your garden. Spraying an infusion of **Marigold Oil** around the house can keep insects away for days.

The easiest way to use Marigolds is, of course, to plant them in flowerpots and set them around the house, enjoying the beautiful colors and the lack of insects.

Also, for the garden, strategically placed Marigold plants can help reduce the occurrence of **Beetles** and **Aphids**.

MINT

Mint, besides being flavorful and having a unique and pleasing odor, is a natural repellant of such insects as **Ants, Mosquitos** and **Flies**. Plant a little Mint in a pot and use the fresh greens for cooking and at the same tile repel insects.

MUMS or Chrysanthemums

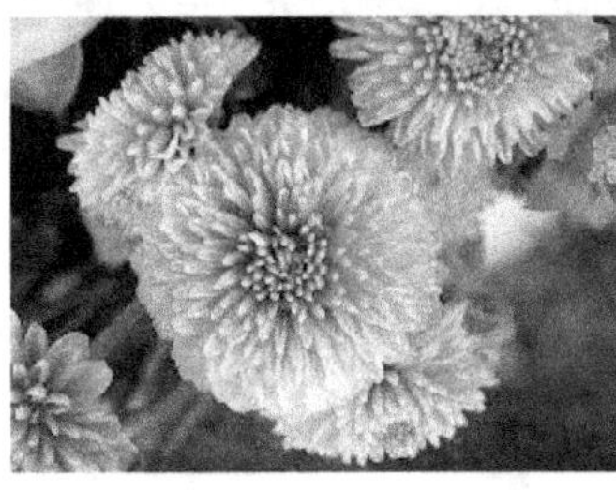

The numerous aromatic sub-species of the Chrysanthemum plant are also excellent mosquito repellants.

The valuable thing about Mums, other than their beauty as a colorful ornamental plant is the fact that the blossoms have a natural chemical compound called *pyrethrins*.

It's the female mosquito who bites people and draws blood. And, this compound can inhibit the female mosquito from biting animals.

So, having a few potted Mums around will cut down your chances of being bitten by mosquitos.

ROSEMARY

The Rosemary plant is a hearty one that will produce for you year round, especially in warmer climates. The evergreen leaves not only add a great flavor to many foods but the aroma of Rosemary is purported to repel **Mosquitos** and several other pest insects.

SUNFLOWERS

The Sunflower is a popular plant that provides beautiful large yellow and black blooms but it is usually planted for its seeds, which are very nutritious.

Sunflowers draw over 120 species of insects. By planting them Sunflowers a good distance away from your garden, you can reduce these insects' damage to your garden.

Other INSECT REPELLANT Tricks

There is another level of Pest control, for insects and also for animal pests that can be quite effective for the gardener who wants to avoid using chemicals on their garden.

GARDEN DECOYS

These simple devices have been used for centuries to drive away garden pests.

 Pests like **Mice, Chipmunks, Squirrels, Rabbits, Deer, Crows** and many other animals that can attack and destroy your garden crop.

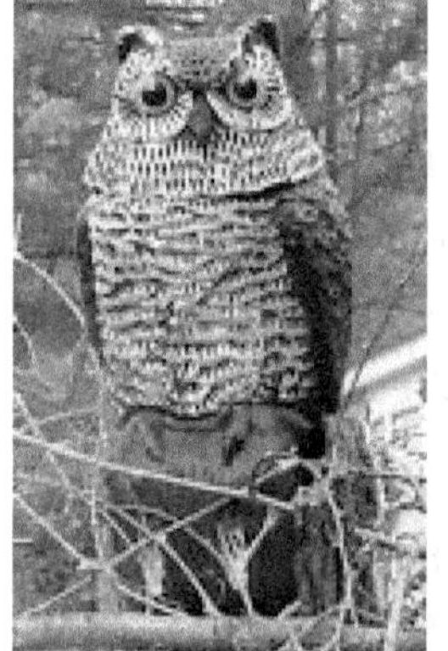

They can often be driven or scared away with certain types of such decoys if they look realistic enough.

Using a **Scarecrow** or using fake predatory birds like **Owls, Hawks** and others will all help scare pests away.

By placing these relatively cheap decoys in and around your garden they will often scare such garden destroyers away from your crops.

PHEROMONE TRAPS

These are simple plastic traps for insects that are designed to trap or contain an insect. Pheromone chemicals can be placed inside these traps that enhance the urge for the insects to reproduce.

the soil until the August/September time of year living on the roots, shoots and even the leaves of many different plants.

At this Larvae stage, they are voracious pests that can quickly destroy a number of garden crops.

CRICKET

The common Cricket is a nocturnal insect that resembles a grasshopper, with similar bodies to the Field Cricket seen here.

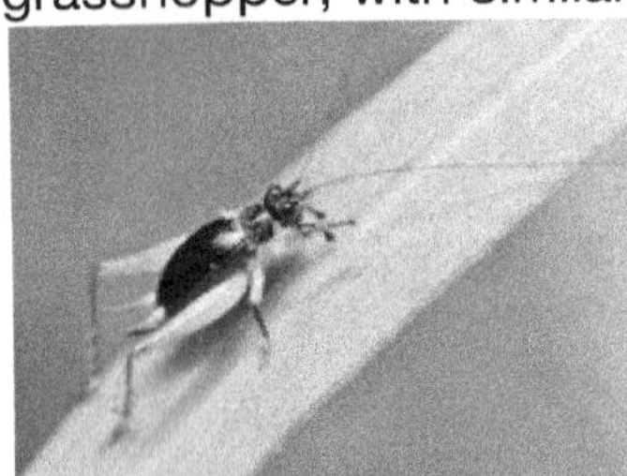

The female can lay as many as 200 eggs at a time that hatch in the spring season.

Some varieties can repeat this process as often as twice a month.

The hatched eggs are destructive pests to farmers, as their preferred foods to eat are young plant seedlings.

Mix Molasses with water in a 1 to 10 ratio and set it in a bowl. The Crickets will be drawn by the sweet smell and then they will drown in the water.

CUTWORM

Cutworms are not actually worms but are Moths in the caterpillar stage of their development.

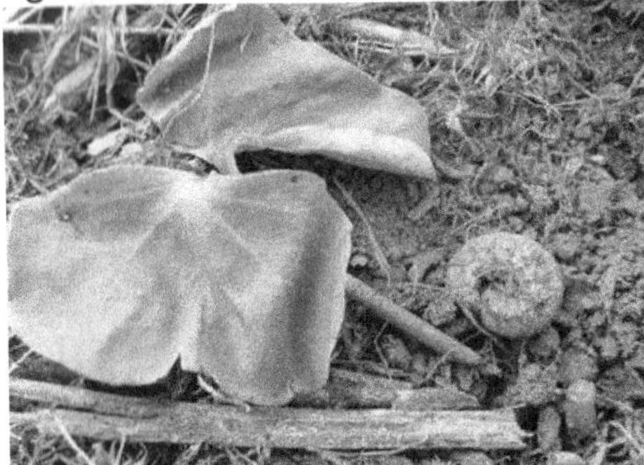

They live in the soil, come out at night and eat plants at the stem level just above the ground.

Cutworms are a very destructive garden pest that can quickly wipe out a large portion of a farmers crops, if they are not controlled quickly.

One eco-friendly method to control cutworm damage is to place paper wrappings around the stems of your garden plants at the ground level.

This layer will keep the cutworms away from the stem of the plant and will eventually rot and not damage the plant as it grows.

Once inside the traps, the insects cannot get out and they eventually die. There are such traps available for over 100 different types of garden pests, mostly varieties of worms and moths.

PLANTING FLOWERS

When strategically between rows of your garden, specifically some of the flowers mentioned in this chapter that Insects and even some wild animals dislike, will reduce the number of some of the insects that could attack your garden.

ROW COVERS

These are made of a light porous plastic and placed over the newly plowed and shaped rows in your garden. Using these can keep many flying insects away from your more susceptible garden plants that you place in cut holes in the material.

STERILITY SPRAYS,

Many of these sprays are made of safe chemicals are capable, when sprayed on your garden, of causing the invading insects to become sterile and not reproduce.

Using these sprays regularly over several years will reduce the population of these garden-ravaging pests.

DIATOMACEOUS Earth

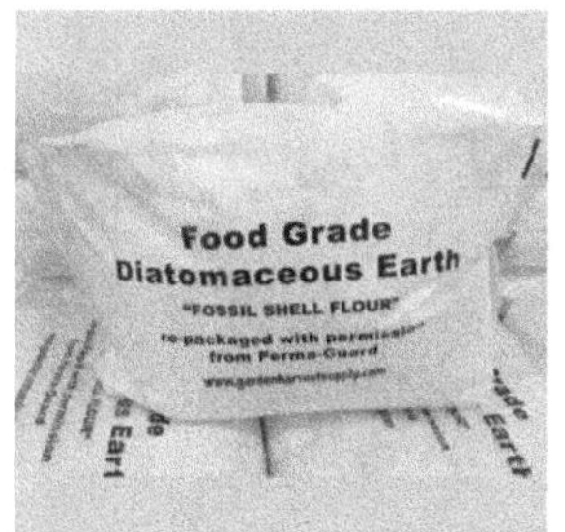

This is a different kind of Pest Control. This product is actually a microscopic fossil with jagged shell edges. It is used by spreading it around the base of crop plants and as a perimeter around the garden.

Any soft-bodied insects will get cut and even torn when they try to crawl over this special kind of dirt.

It can be used around your food plants and later it can be worked into the soil to kill those grubs and other below-the -surface insects.

This special kind of soil can work for you in your garden for several years before you have to apply more.

Garden INSECT PESTS and their ENEMIES

Over the long history of the Planet Earth there have been two dominate species that thrived. First there were the Dinosaurs in all of their grand variety, but for whatever eventually becomes the final reason, they became extinct and the next dominant species has risen to its age of greatness, the human species.

Over this long period of time, each species has had to live in conjunction with the mighty Insect. Each variety of insects is highly specialized in their life cycle, especially their preferred temperate zone and foods.

Some Insects we admire and we even enjoy the fruits of their labors both directly and indirectly such as Honey from Bees and pollinated flowers of fruit plants. But, most insects are big problems for humans and destructive to the production of many of our foods.

In this chapter you will see a listing of a number of the insects that are considered garden pests. But, also there will be a list of other insects that live on certain of these Insect Pests.

Learn how to use them properly and you will improve your garden output naturally and avoid using those deadly insect repellants on the market.

INSECT PESTS:

There are literally hundreds of insect pests that can attack and destroy your garden plants. Even the gardener with a small crop of their favorite foods can have their garden plants devastated by these hungry and aggressive little pests.

Below you will find valuable information on some of the most **common Pest Insects** that you will often find in your garden.

APHIDS

Aphids are pest insects that range in size of between one and ten millimeters in length.

And, as a group, they are the most destructive of Insect pests to home gardeners and even other commercial farmers.

Many Aphids are specialized and eat only one plant species, b

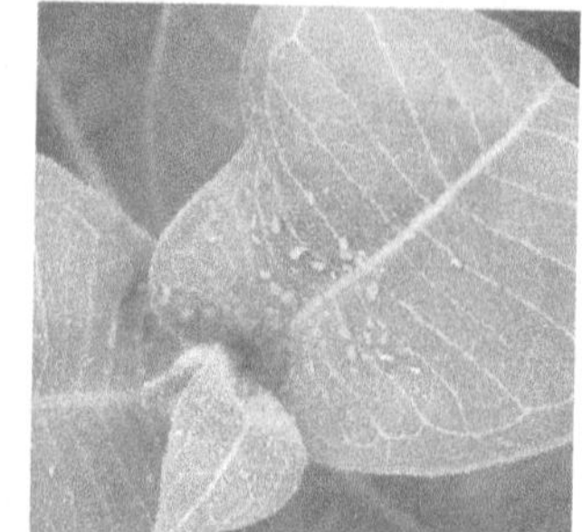

there are some who are destructive threats to multiple types of garden plants.

There are a number of insects that f on Aphids, but many of these can b attacked themselves by ants if any around.

Ants will actually protect Aphids fro other insects to get the "honeydew" that the Aphids produce.

Neem Oil is an organic pesticide that is popularly used to cont Aphids on garden plants.

BEETLE

Beetles are insects with a hard shell and usually have two sets wings.

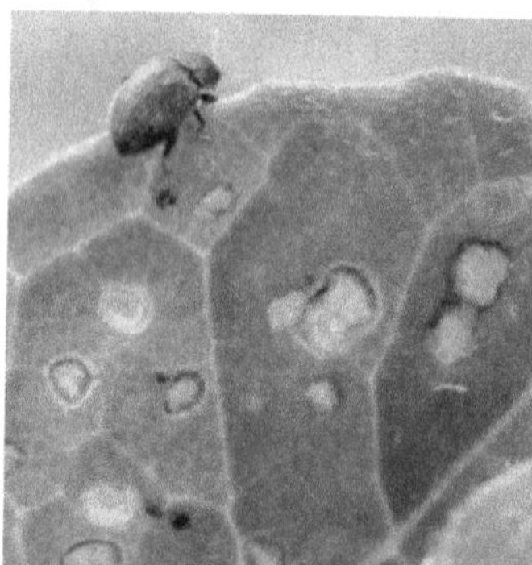

There are actually hundreds of varie of Beetles but several varieties are destructive to certain crops.

One of the more common varieties on farms and in gardens is the Flea Beetle, seen here.

The **Japanese Beetle**, the **Grapevi Hoplia** and the **June Beetle** are examples of the most destructive Beetles that farmer must contend w

Because they actually fly to the plants they eat, using hanging t containing a liquid combination of Honey to Water in a 1-to-10 will capture many of these pests efficiently.

CRANE FLY

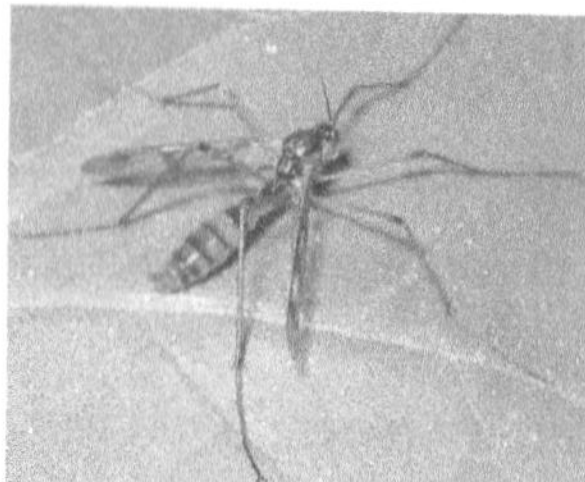

The Crane Fly grows fast and can be u 2-1/2 inches long resembling giant mosquitos but at this adult stage they c eat leaves.

And, at this stage they do not bite like t Mosquitos they resemble.

Their Larvae hide out in the upper layers

Once inside the traps, the insects cannot get out and they eventually die. There are such traps available for over 100 different types of garden pests, mostly varieties of worms and moths.

PLANTING FLOWERS

When strategically between rows of your garden, specifically some of the flowers mentioned in this chapter that Insects and even some wild animals dislike, will reduce the number of some of the insects that could attack your garden.

ROW COVERS

These are made of a light porous plastic and placed over the newly plowed and shaped rows in your garden. Using these can keep many flying insects away from your more susceptible garden plants that you place in cut holes in the material.

STERILITY SPRAYS,

Many of these sprays are made of safe chemicals are capable, when sprayed on your garden, of causing the invading insects to become sterile and not reproduce.

Using these sprays regularly over several years will reduce the population of these garden-ravaging pests.

DIATOMACEOUS Earth

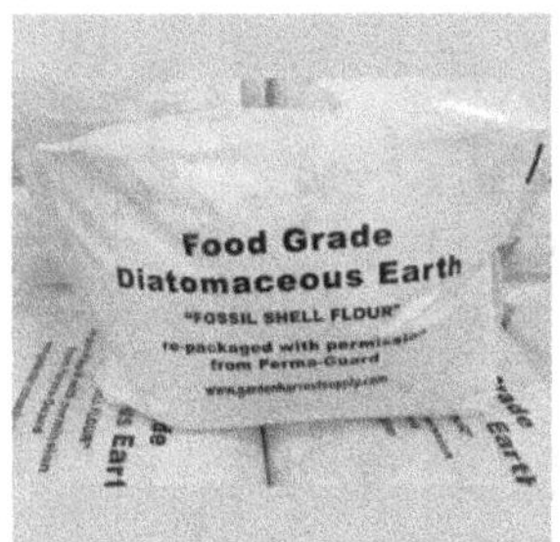

This is a different kind of Pest Control. This product is actually a microscopic fossil with jagged shell edges. It is used by spreading it around the base of crop plants and as a perimeter around the garden.

Any soft-bodied insects will get cut and even torn when they try to crawl over this special kind of dirt.

It can be used around your food plants and later it can be worked into the soil to kill those grubs and other below-the -surface insects.

This special kind of soil can work for you in your garden for several years before you have to apply more.

Garden INSECT PESTS and their ENEMIES

Over the long history of the Planet Earth there have been two dominate species that thrived. First there were the Dinosaurs in all of their grand variety, but for whatever eventually becomes the final reason, they became extinct and the next dominant species has risen to its age of greatness, the human species.

Over this long period of time, each species has had to live in conjunction with the mighty Insect. Each variety of insects is highly specialized in their life cycle, especially their preferred temperate zone and foods.

Some Insects we admire and we even enjoy the fruits of their labors both directly and indirectly such as Honey from Bees and pollinated flowers of fruit plants. But, most insects are big problems for humans and destructive to the production of many of our foods.

In this chapter you will see a listing of a number of the insects that are considered garden pests. But, also there will be a list of other insects that live on certain of these Insect Pests.

Learn how to use them properly and you will improve your garden output naturally and avoid using those deadly insect repellants on the market.

INSECT PESTS:

There are literally hundreds of insect pests that can attack and destroy your garden plants. Even the gardener with a small crop of their favorite foods can have their garden plants devastated by these hungry and aggressive little pests.

Below you will find valuable information on some of the most **common Pest Insects** that you will often find in your garden.

APHIDS

Aphids are pest insects that range in size of between one and ten millimeters in length.

And, as a group, they are the most destructive of Insect pests to home gardeners and even other commercial farmers.

Many Aphids are specialized and eat only one plant species, but

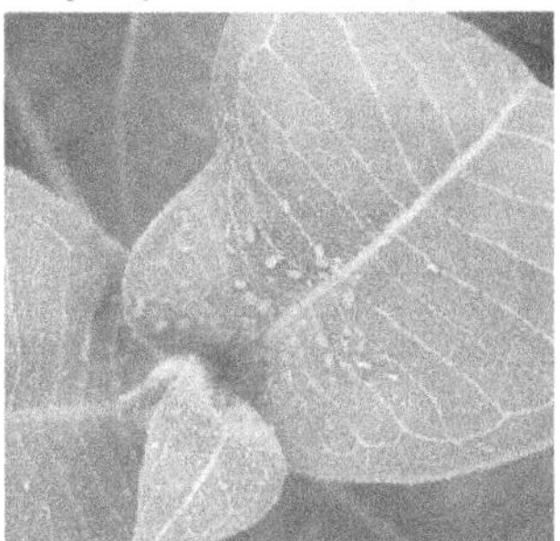

there are some who are destructive threats to multiple types of garden plants.

There are a number of insects that feed on Aphids, but many of these can be attacked themselves by ants if any are around.

Ants will actually protect Aphids from other insects to get the "honeydew" that the Aphids produce.

Neem Oil is an organic pesticide that is popularly used to control Aphids on garden plants.

BEETLE

Beetles are insects with a hard shell and usually have two sets of wings.

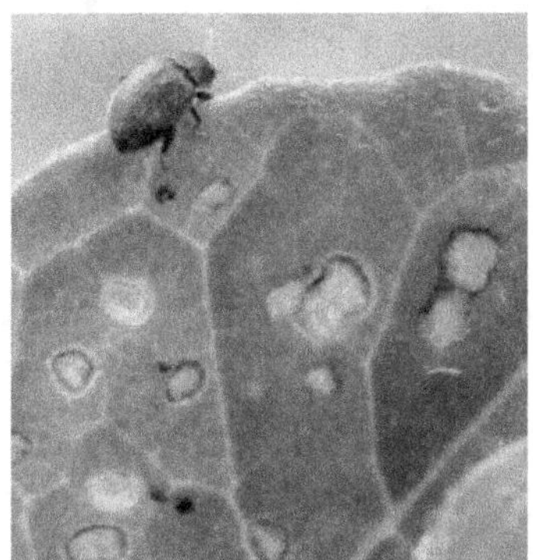

There are actually hundreds of varieties of Beetles but several varieties are very destructive to certain crops.

One of the more common varieties found on farms and in gardens is the Flea Beetle, seen here.

The **Japanese Beetle**, the **Grapevine Hoplia** and the **June Beetle** are examples of the most destructive Beetles that farmer must contend with.

Because they actually fly to the plants they eat, using hanging traps containing a liquid combination of Honey to Water in a 1-to-10 ratio will capture many of these pests efficiently.

CRANE FLY

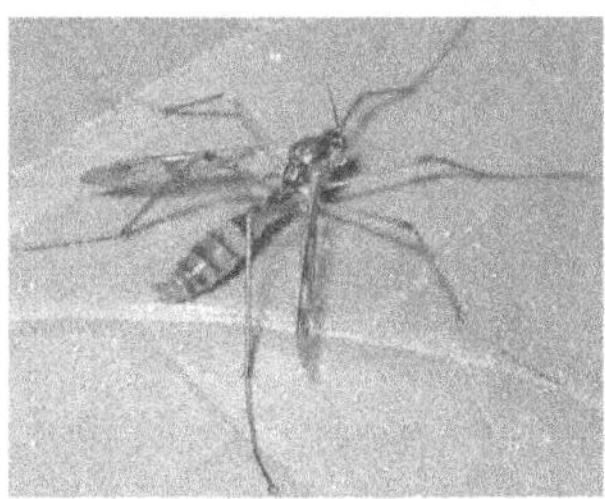

The Crane Fly grows fast and can be up to 2-1/2 inches long resembling giant mosquitos but at this adult stage they only eat leaves.

And, at this stage they do not bite like the Mosquitos they resemble.

Their Larvae hide out in the upper layers of

Donald W Bobbitt

the soil until the August/September time of year living on the roots, shoots and even the leaves of many different plants.

At this Larvae stage, they are voracious pests that can quickly destroy a number of garden crops.

CRICKET

The common Cricket is a nocturnal insect that resembles a grasshopper, with similar bodies to the Field Cricket seen here.

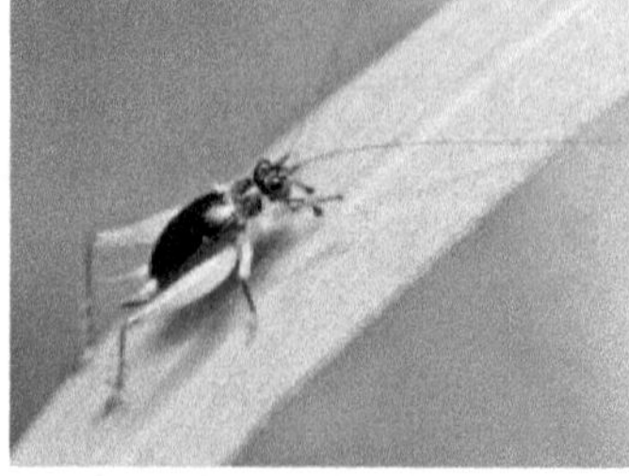

The female can lay as many as 200 eggs at a time that hatch in the spring season.

Some varieties can repeat this process as often as twice a month.

The hatched eggs are destructive pests to farmers, as their preferred foods to eat are young plant seedlings.

Mix Molasses with water in a 1 to 10 ratio and set it in a bowl. The Crickets will be drawn by the sweet smell and then they will drown in the water.

CUTWORM

Cutworms are not actually worms but are Moths in the caterpillar stage of their development.

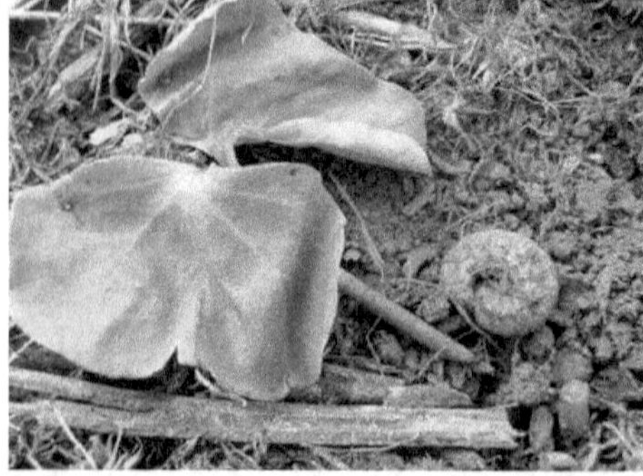

They live in the soil, come out at night and eat plants at the stem level just above the ground.

Cutworms are a very destructive garden pest that can quickly wipe out a large portion of a farmers crops, if they are not controlled quickly.

One eco-friendly method to control cutworm damage is to place paper wrappings around the stems of your garden plants at the ground level.

This layer will keep the cutworms away from the stem of the plant and will eventually rot and not damage the plant as it grows.

FUNGUS GNAT

The adult Fungus Gnat actually lives on Fungus, as its name

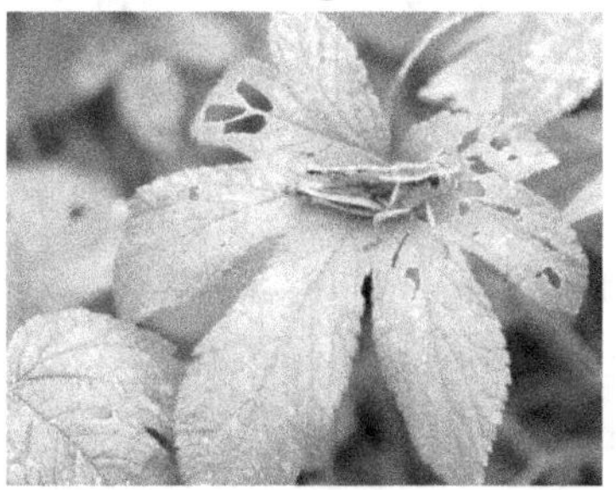

implies, but, in the larvae stage, they will feed on a number of young garden plants causing flesh wounds to the shoots.

These wounds in the young shoots as well as mature plant stalks allow access points for the growth of plant killing pathogens that can spread and

kill the infected garden plant.

GRASSHOPPER

Grasshoppers are of a grouping of insects that have mandibles and they will tear the leaves of the plants that they eat.

In large numbers, they can be devastating to crops and their preferred foods are; grasses, leaves of just about any plant and also cereal crops.

For the home gardener, even a small number of grasshoppers can harm the vitality of your garden plants.

GRUB

If you have a patch of rich soil, it is likely that sooner or later you will

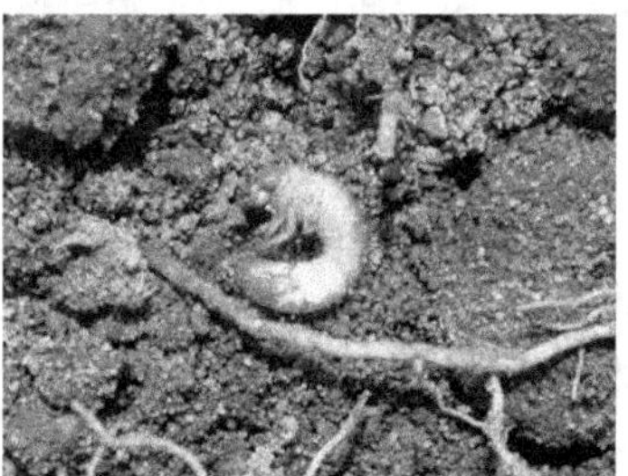

find Grubs just below the surface.

Most of the Grubs found in gardens are actually the larvae if such insects as Beetles, Scarabs, June Bugs and Japanese Beetles.

Grubs are a double threat to gardens.

In the larvae stage they attack and eat

plant roots and then once they hatch, they will eat the greenery of the plants.

LEAF HOPPER

Leaf Hoppers are very small insects that can destroy a plant with the pathogens it often carries.

 They feed by sucking the sap from many different plants, even from some small shrubs and trees.

Donald W Bobbitt

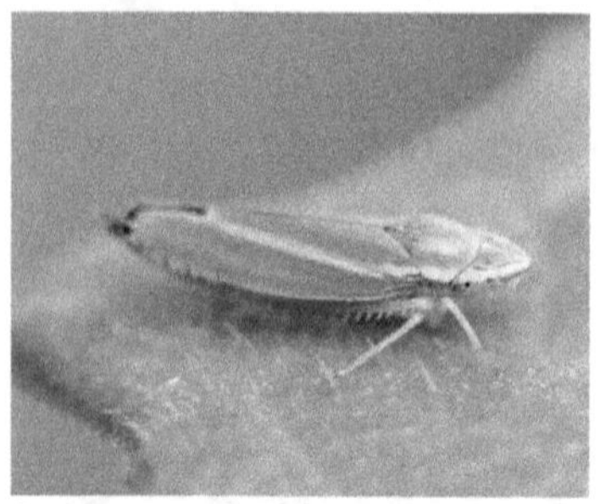

The problem with these pests is that they not only feed but can also carry a plant pathogen that infects many of the plants they feed on.

These pathogens include various viruses and fungi that eventually end up infecting and destroying the plant.

Leaf Hoppers are quite mobile and can find and devastate a garden crop quickly, so a fast response is necessary when you spot them.

LEAF BLISTER MITES

Leaf Blister Mites are microscopic insects that feed on the leaves of such fruit trees as Apples and Peaches.

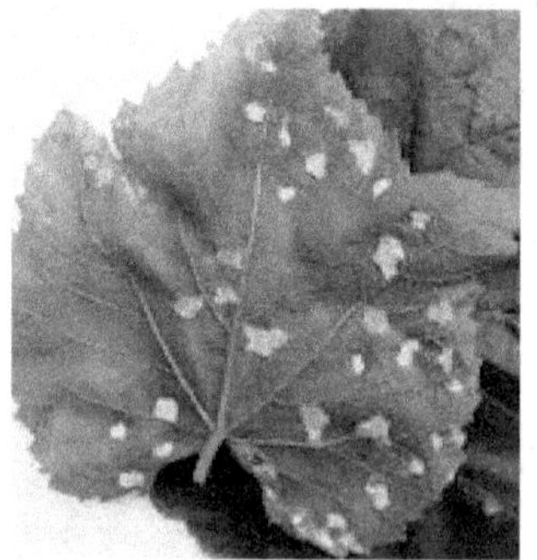

Typically, they will generate a small blister of a material that hardens on the leaves and the fruit of a plant.

This blister then gives them protection from predators and then they are able to move in and out of the blisters to feed on the leaves of the plant.

These miniature pests are often found living on abandoned or untreated fruit trees that have not been maintained properly.

MEALYBUGS

These small pests, called Mealy Bugs, are among the most

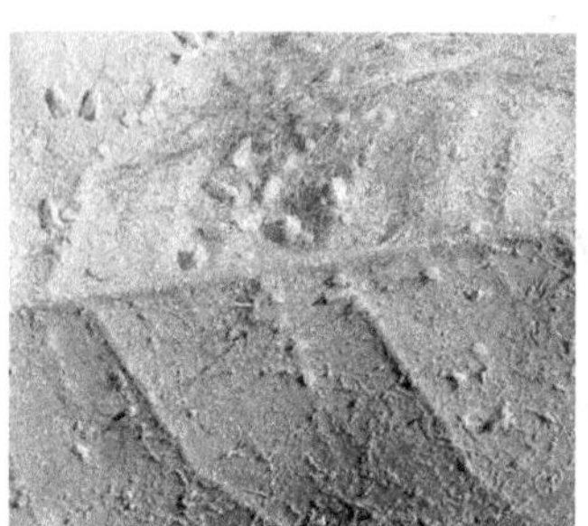

destructive of garden plant eaters. They prosper around the world in warm moist climates.

They have unprotected (no scales) bodies and the female lives on the sap of numerous different plants, specifically Citrus plants and various houseplants and greenhouse plants.

They attach themselves to plants and secrete a waxy substance for protection while they feed on the juices of the plant.

64

These pests often carry plant pathogens that can destroy the plants that they are feeding on.

Ladybird beetles feed on mealy bugs. A 50/50 solution of Isopropyl alcohol and household detergent can be used to destroy Mealy Bugs. The alcohol will melt the waxy covering and the household cleanser will kill the bugs.

MOTHS

There are over 160,000 species of Moths and most species are nocturnal.

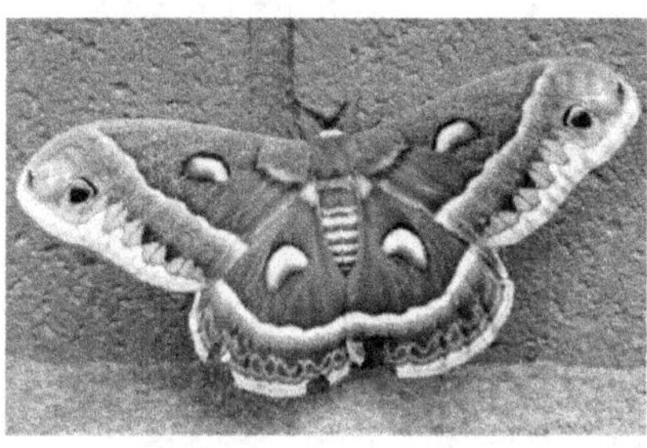

The Moth larvae, in its cocoon stage, lives in the ground until it emerges as an adult moth.

They are, by nature, in both the larvae and adult stages, devourers of numerous plants and their foliage. The Gypsy Moth in both the larvae and the adult stages are devastating to many crops specifically, fruit farm crops.

Moths are pests that must be controlled to protect crops. Such animals as bats, owls, other birds, lizards, rats and even dogs and cats will eat moths.

POTATO BEETLE

The Colorado Potato Beetle is an insect that can devastate some crops. They are less than a half-inch long with bright yellow bodies and have ten brown stripes on their backs.

It is one of a number of specialized pests, of the beetle family, that attack and devour the leaves and shoots of potato plants.

Even though they are known for their damage to potato plants, these pests will also eat eggplants, tomato plants, pepper plants and even the plants of petunias.

They feed on the foliage of a plant and eat until the leaves are skeletonized.

Over time these pests have developed resistance to the numerous insecticides used on them, including the deadly DDT. There are certain ground beetles that feed on Potato beetles and there are certain fungi that feed on them which can be grown and used.

Donald W Bobbitt

ROOTWORM

Rootworms, particularly the corn rootworms shown here, feed on the roots of corn plants.

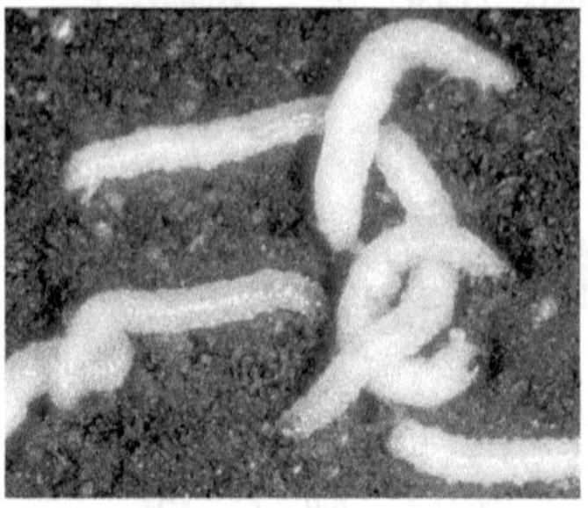

In the larvae stage they have six pairs of legs that are not visible to the naked eye and they have a brown head and a brown marking on their last abdominal segment.

In the adult stage, they are yellow in color and have a brown stripe on each wing cover.

They feed on the corn silk, pollen and kernels of the ear of corn.

Rootworms can destroy a significant part of a crop if left unmanaged.

SCALES

Scales are round shaped small insects that attach themselves to a plant and live on the plants sap.

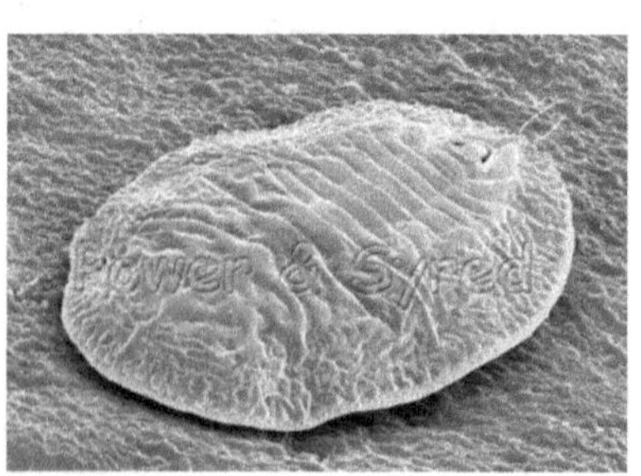

Once they attach themselves to a plant, they protect themselves with a waxy outer shell that often also protects them from insecticides.

Scales attack the leaves and plant stems but rarely the fruit of the plant.

Horticultural oils are often used to kill (suffocate) them.

SPIDER MITES

These pests live on the underside of plant leaves and usually spin a web around themselves for protection.

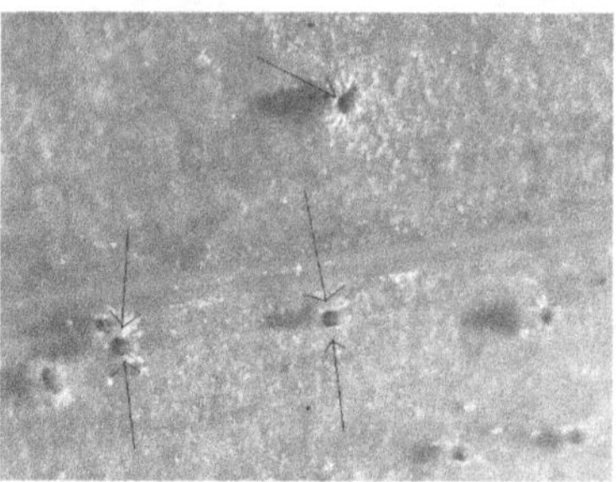

They are known to feed on over 200 species of plants, specifically beans, corn, potatoes, peppers, strawberries, tomatoes, and cannabis.

The female can lay up to 20 eggs a day and live up to 4-weeks.

66

This life cycle allow them to adapt quickly to pesticide varieties.

WEEVILS

The Weevil insect is typically less than ¼-inch long and the female

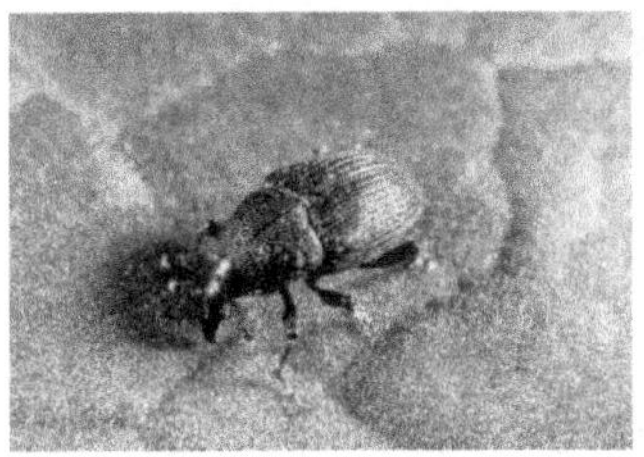

lays large numbers of eggs, so early recognition and control is imperative to protect your crops.

The Weevil is a type of Beetle that is often found eating such crop foods as **Cereals, Grains, Nuts**, and even **Cotton.**

And, they can often be found in dry stored foods such as Flour.

GOOD INSECTS, that eat BAD Insects

The smart gardener knows that there are some insects they want to see in their gardens and yards. These insects actually eat and control the population of certain other insects and here are a few of them;

CRAB SPIDERS:

Crab or Flower Spiders (Selenopids) live on flowering plants and

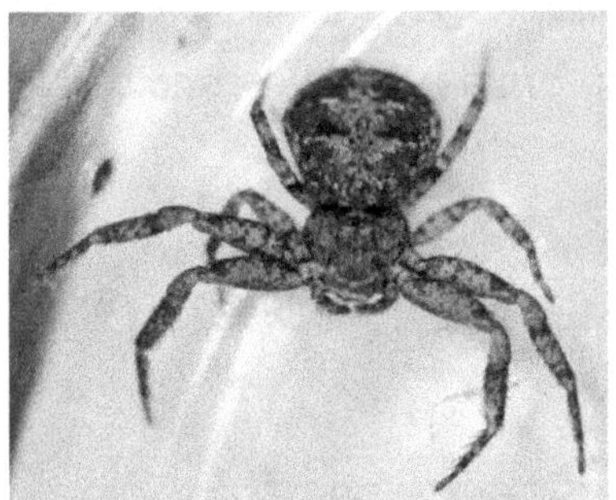

they eat the insects that the flowers of the plant draw.

A large female Crab Spider requires a lot of food to product healthy eggs.

In Florida there is a very colorful spider that is called colloquially the Crab Spider whose real name is The Spiny Back Weaver.

It has an outer shell that is usually white with black and bright red spikes.

This variety is actually poisonous but it will usually, at the most, just give a human an itch if bitten.

GREEN LACEWINGS:

The Green Lacewing can be from as small as 6mm to a large as 50-mm in some tropical areas.

Its body is generally bright green to brownish-green in color while their large wings are translucent with visible veins.

They also have hearing organs in the wings and can hear a bat's ultrasonic calls.

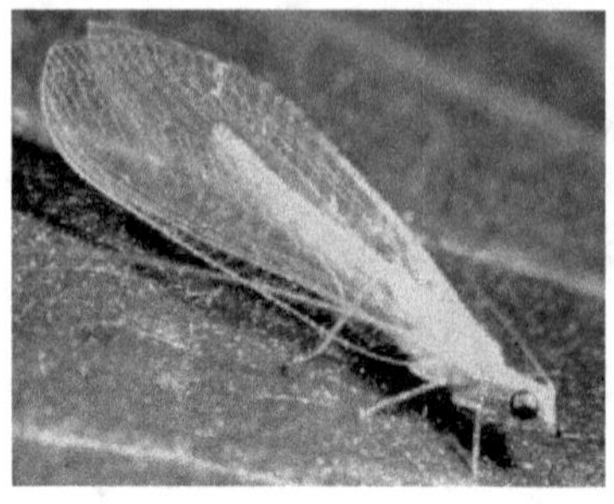

It is an insect that feeds on a number of other insects, specifically the soft-bodied ones including **Aphids, Mites, Thrips, Leafhoppers** and **Whitefly**.

They also eat the larvae, or caterpillars of **Beetles, Pest Moths** and **Mealy bugs,** among others.

HOVERFLIES:

Hoverflies, also known as **Flower Flies** or **Syrphid Flies** and can be recognized because they have only one pair of wings.

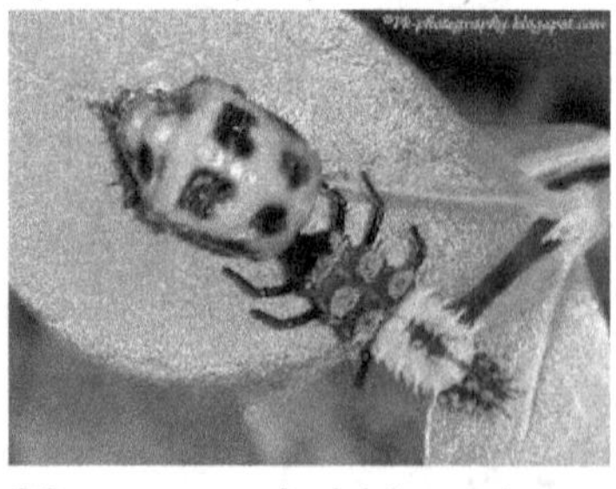

While in their larvae stage, Hoverflies are great to have around for controlling such pests as **Aphids, Caterpillars, Scales** and **Thrips**.

In the Adult stage, they are great plant pollinators as well as voracious pest insect eaters.

LADYBUGS:

Ladybugs are not only beautiful little insects, but more importantly for gardeners, they also thrive on eating other pest insect, specifically Aphids.

Ladybugs are natural predators to soft-bodied pests such as; **Aphids, Leaf Hoppers, Mealy Bugs, Mites, Scales, Spider Mites**, various larvae and other soft bodied insects

An adult Ladybug is a prolific eater of Aphids and can consume as many as 80 or more Aphids a day.

Ladybugs also help in plant pollination, so, enjoy the beauty of the Ladybug and the knowledge that they are ridding your garden of those destructive Aphids.

MINUTE POWER BUG:

The Minute Power Bug is only about 1/8-inch long and is a black bug with white markings at the base of its wings.

This useful insect feeds on a number of pests, including; **Aphids, Chinch bugs, Springtails, Thrips** and the eggs of; **Corn Earworms, Spider Mites** and **Whiteflies**.

NEMATODES:

Encouraging the growth of Nematodes in your soil will give the gardener protection from a wide variety of Insect pests.

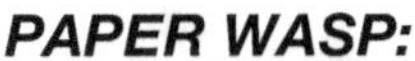

These pests include; **Cutworms, Flea larvae, Fungus Gnat, Grubs, Ladybugs, Rootworms, Spider Mites** and **Weevils**, among others.

Nematodes are actually microscopic worm-like creatures that live in your soil, year round and they thrive on the insects listed above, among others, when they are living in the soil.

PAPER WASP:

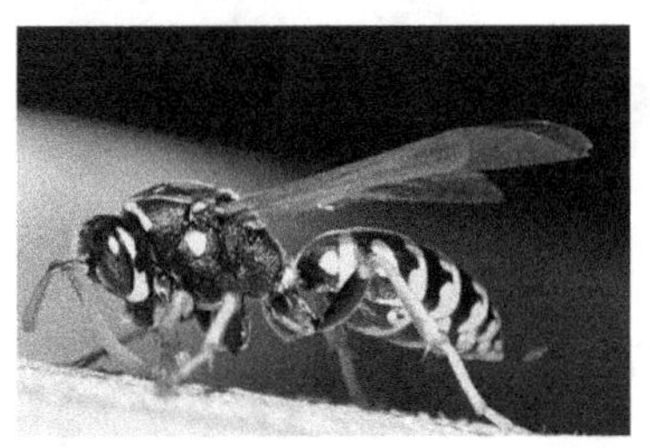

The Paper Wasp is also known as the **Umbrella Wasp**.

It is a useful insect for farmers and gardeners alike because of the variety of garden pest insects that it eats.

The Paper Wasp feeds on the Caterpillars of a number of pest insects including **Army Worms, Corn Earworms,** and **Hornworms**, among others.

PRAYING MANTIS:

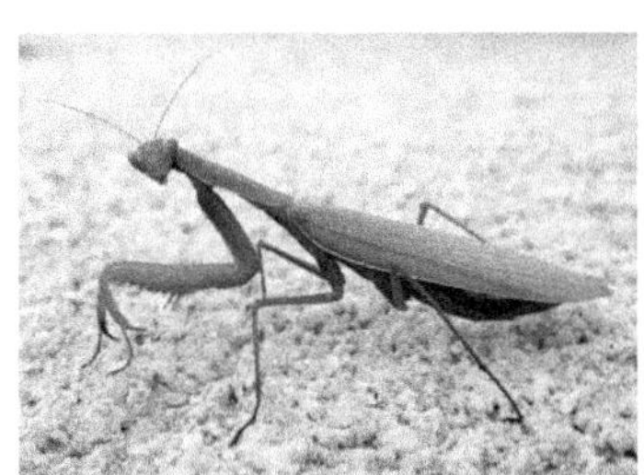

The Praying Mantis is not only an impressive and unique insect to look at, it's also a voracious consumer of a number of different Pest Insects that attack a gardeners crops.

When you do see a Praying Mantis in or near your garden, do not kill or even bother it.

The Praying Mantis are big eaters and their favorite meals are such pest insects as; **Beetles, Crane Flies, Crickets, Flies, Grasshoppers, Mosquitos, Moths** and **Wasps**, among others.

STOCKPILING FOODS to Save

Stockpiling certain foods can save you a lot of money as well as provide fresh and safe food stores for you and your family, in emergency situations.

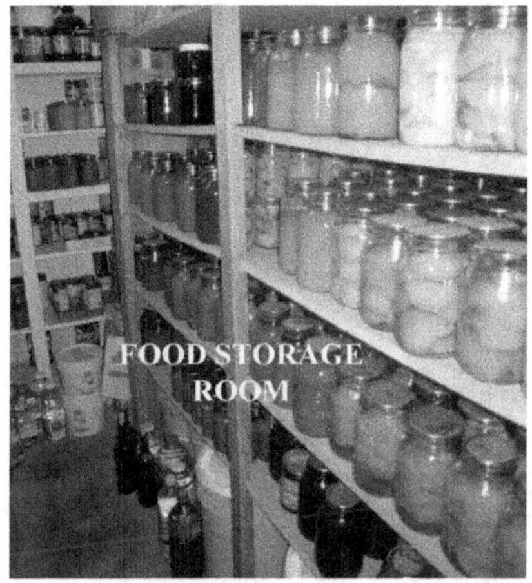

We have all heard about and even seen references to sites that will sell the serious survivalist large containers of packaged foods to be stored for those radical potential emergency situations.

But, anyone can stockpile decent quantities of foods.

A stockpile of just two weeks worth of foods for you and your family can actually takes up a relatively small amount of space.

And if you stockpile smartly you can not only save money on your grocery bills, but, at the same time, you will have a significant food resource for such things as; extended power outages, weather catastrophes, natural disasters, etcetera.

A Stockpile Pantry

Every home has a pantry of sorts where you normally store your canned foods, spices and other dry goods until you need to use them.

Typically, this type of pantry includes one or two of each item and they are kept there until you need them over the next week or so.

But, if you are truly frugal, you can also establish a special area in your home for stockpiling larger quantities of those same great food deals; that is separate from your regular and often limited kitchen pantry.

For the small-scale stockpile you can simply modify an unused closet with a few extra shelves or if you are a more serious stockpiler, you can fill a larger area in a basement or heated and cooled garage with shelves.

If your garage is not heated, try keeping your foods in large plastic tubs with sealable tops.

The basic requirement for storing foods is that the area used for storage be cool and dry.

Buy Cheap and Store the extra:

The purchasing process is very easy. You just need to take advantage of two things, sales and coupons.

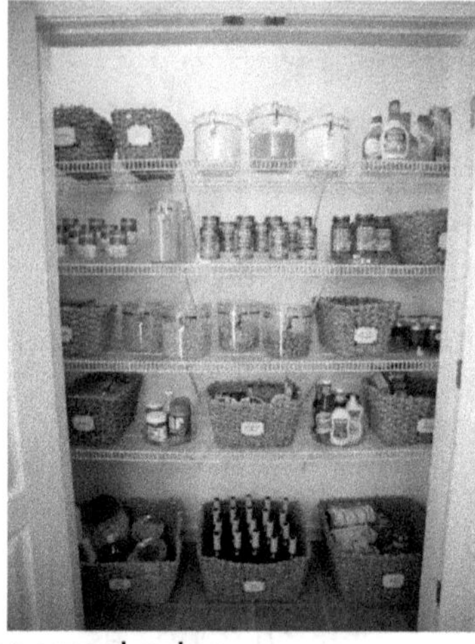

If you start thinking about your groceries as commodities that you will always need, rather than just something you need for next week's dinner then you will realize that buying sale items, often even in larger volumes, will save you significant money.

For instance, you may not even need any canned beans at the time but as you walk down the supermarket aisle you might see that they are having a sale on your favorite beans at half their normal price.

If you pick up, say six cans at this great price rather than your normal one can and take them home for your stockpile pantry, over time you will be eating your favorite beans at half their normal cost.

For instance, say that the normal price for a can of beans is $1.00 per can so by buying six cans at $0.50 per can ends up being a savings of $3.00. Multiply this by maybe twenty of your most used food items and you will have realized a significant savings by stockpiling just these few items.

Another way to save big while stockpiling is to make a habit of scanning through the coupons in your newspaper and pulling the ones that offer a good savings on your favorite food items.

On your next trip to your supermarket, purchase several of these discounted items and place them into your special pantry when the savings is large enough to matter.

By just using these two ways of saving, your pantry will soon be filled with great foods that you can consume at your leisure, knowing that you have saved some significant money on each item.

Items you can easily Stockpile

Of course, everyone's tastes are different, but below is a list of some of the most commonly consumed foods by families that also store very well:

Canned Liquids – Canned, Broths, Condensed Milk, Canned Soups, Canned Vegetables

Canned Vegetables – Artichoke Hearts, Beans, Corn, Green Beans, Peas, Pickles, Tomatoes and Beans in general.

Canned Sauces – Barbecue Sauces, Tomato Sauces, Chili, canned gravies

Canned Meats – Beef and other canned red meats, canned Chicken, Corned Beef, Salmon, Tuna and other canned fish.

Canned Fruits – Apples, Oranges, Peaches, Pears, Pineapple, Fruit Cocktail

Canned Condiments – Catsup, Jams, Mayonnaise, Peanut Butter, Salad Dressings

Cooking Oils – Vegetable Oils, Olive Oil, Corn Oil

Dry Goods – Cereals, Flour, Corn Meal, Rice, Dried Beans, Crackers, Coffee, Pasta, Tea Bags

Dry Vegetables – Dried Garlic, Dried Onions, Dried Hot Peppers, Dried Fruits, Dried Herbs and Spices such a Rosemary and Dill.

Pickled Foods – Pickled Cucumbers, Fish, Squash, Hot Peppers, Onions, Eggs, Sausages.

Salt Cured Meats – Salt Fish, Salt Pork, Salt Beef and other red meats.

Inventory Control

One thing that you absolutely must do if you are going to stockpile foods is come up with a way to keep up with the storage dates and how many you have of each item.

You do not want to put something away in your stockpile and when you do get around to using it, find out that it has spoiled. Nor do you want to look onto your shelves and find dozens of an item that you only use 3-4 of a year.

Keep in mind that even canned goods should be consumed within twelve months of purchase. Dried goods, if stored properly, should be consumed within three to six months of being purchased or if labeled with a "**consume by date**" or "**sell by date**", within a couple of weeks of that date.

The simplest way to manage your stockpile is to use a permanent marker and label (try a cheap masking tape for a label) every can and package with the date that you put it into your stockpile.

Then, as you look for an item to use, you can quickly check and use the oldest dated can or package. By rotating your stockpile you will be eating good foods and saving a lot of money.

Everyone should use the stockpiling philosophy to one degree or another for savings on your food purchases. You might be someone who just wants to concentrate on saving a few dollars.

Or you can be someone who wants the added security of knowing that you have one or two or even more weeks of food supplies stored away, just in case you might need them.

Be aware of what you are stockpiling. Often you can have such a large quantity of an item that it becomes a problem, For instance, lotions are notorious for going bad after a while in storage. And, often, if you have a multiple year supply of something it could be taking up valuable storage space that you might use for yet another item.

Regardless of your reasoning, with careful management, stockpiling can work for you.

How to Store ROOT VEGETABLES

Root Vegetables such as potatoes, carrots, turnips, rutabagas and beets, among others are delicious and nutritional foods that are planted and raised in many gardens.

The problem for many farmers is the fact that these are seasonal foods and people need ways to store them for use in the colder winter season, if possible.

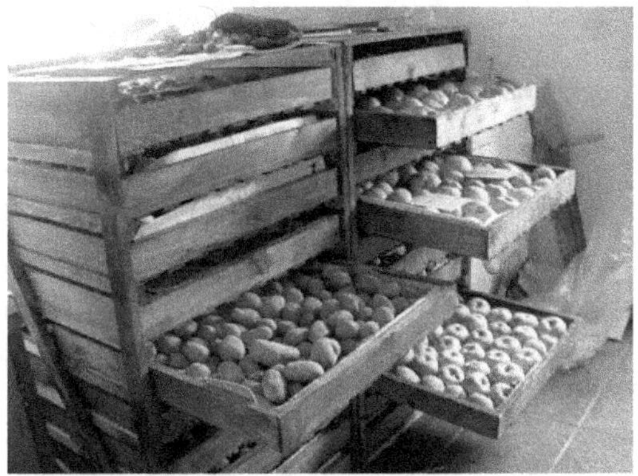

Long ago, a farmer would have a springhouse on his property that was ideal for storing certain foods.

A springhouse was just that. If there were a spring on your property, you would clean out the spring and build a small roofed structure over the area.

This way, the springhouse was clean and cool and you still allowed that fresh clean water to flow naturally on to your farm

Your small shed-like structure around the head of the spring was then ideal for storing your foods that the heat might make go bad early, such as milk, butter, eggs and more. This was the precursor to the refrigerator.

The air temperature in the springhouse would always be cool and moist. You could store your butter, milk and fresh vegetables on shelves or even in the water and they would last days longer than being stored in your much hotter home.

And you would usually have a shelf or two reserved for storing any excess root vegetables.

Some farmers would have planned ahead and dug a small cellar under their house for storing their root vegetables, to get the same temperature conditions as in a Spring House.

By using such a controlled and consistent environment and by keep these roots away from the sun; they can often be stored for several months.

You can even use a cool corner of your basement, if you can control the air temperature and the moisture level. You want these roots to stay dormant, thinking that they are still in the ground.

Storing Roots on a Shelf:

If you have an ideal spot, like a springhouse or root cellar, you can just place some ole newspapers on the shelf and then place your root vegetables, in a single layer onto the newspapers for storage.

You can also use straw, peat moss or wood chips on the shelf if they are kept moist, and place your roots on this material.

Storing Roots in Boxes

If you have a large quantity of roots to store, you can use cardboard boxes, lined with newspapers, or the other mentioned materials. Do not over-fill the boxes placing the roots loosely in the box to allow good airflow between them before adding another layer of liner materials and then more roots.

Make sure the cardboard boxes have air holes in them and if not just cut a few 1-inch holes around the sides of the boxes.

Boxes can be stacked, 2 or 3 high, but be sure to give yourself easy access to them so you can check the vegetables regularly.

Managing your Stored Root Vegetables

Once you have your vegetables stored, you need to check them at least weekly. The materials they are stored on must be kept moist so have a spray bottle of water handy.

Check for deteriorating roots each week and remove and use any that look like they may be going soft on you.

Root Vegetables are going to eventually start generating new shoots. This is natural and you just need to monitor them regularly.

At some point, these shoots will be so large that they are robbing the root itself of nutrients and body mass that you will need to start using them.

In summary, store your root vegetables properly and you can enjoy these tasty fruits of your labors through most of the winter months.

Dry Your Own Foods

Drying foods and herbs was once a very popular way to preserve a food that has fallen out of use in modern technical societies.

But drying is still a very efficient way to preserve excess crops of foods, =herbs and even meats for consumption at a later time, especially when heeded in the winter.

Preparation: Most fruits and vegetables should be either; cut into small (typically ½-inch) chunks, or thinly sliced to facilitate the drying process.

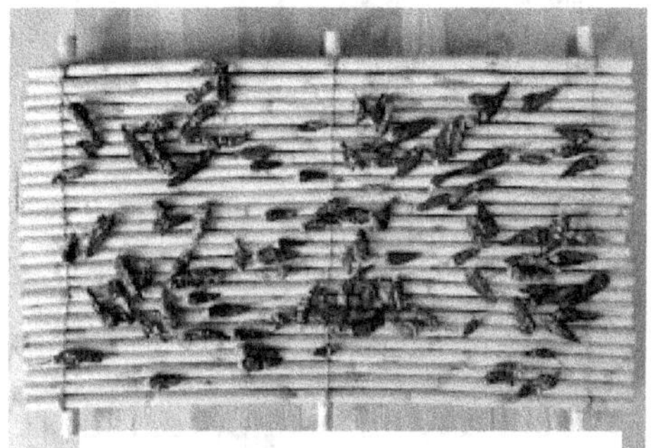

PEPPERS on Drying Rack

Meats are usually sliced and heavily salted if they are to be dried. Some meats are ground up, along with flavorful herbs and spices, as well as salt and then ground up.

The ground meat and spice combination is then mixed well to assure a consistent blend.

Once it is blended well the meat is shaped into thin long strips and laid out on wax paper before drying.

You can brush the meat strips with an acidic solution such as a 75/25 solution of lemon juice and distilled water. This will help preserve the natural color of the food during the drying process.

Be sure to avoid having bones in the meat, as well as seeds and pits in the fruits.

Dehydrators: Today, some people opt for the convenience of electric dehydrators to dry their foods. These specialized machines are fast and efficient tools for the user to dry their foods.

Dehydrators, for individual use, are usually small and somewhat costly to purchase but they almost guarantee success with every batch of food they are used to dry.

Oven Drying: But, if you are going to dry a relatively small quantity of foods, and then only occasionally, you can often do this quite easily in your home oven.

Donald W Bobbitt

Simply prepare your foods to be dried and place them onto a tray with a screen cover. I recommend using a roasting pan with its slotted tray cover in order to drain any excess liquids such as water and fats.

Then you set the oven to a low temperature and just check the drying food every hour until the food drying reaches the state that you want.

Sun Drying: But, it is also easy to use Mother Nature and the sun to dry your excess foods.

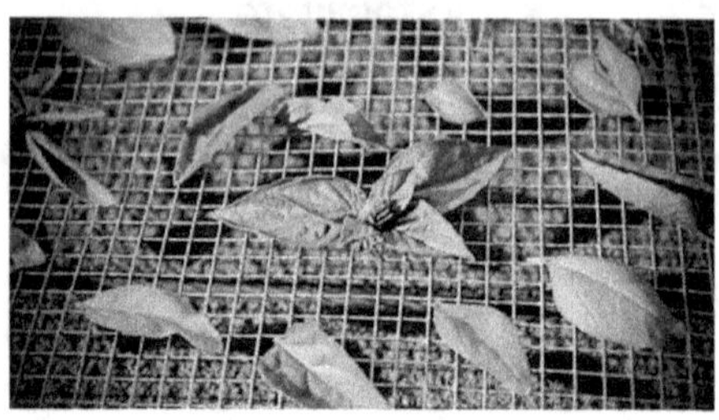

HERB leaves on Air Drying Rack

Just place the foods to be dried onto trays (made of screen, if possible) and cover the food loosely with a plastic wrap or a loose weave cloth to keep the animals and insects away.

Then place the trays in the direct sunlight until the foods have dried properly.

Bring the trays inside for the night or at least cover the trays at night to avoid any rain or dew damage.

It may take days to dry your foods in the sun but otherwise, once the foods have dried properly, store these nutritionally rich foods in containers for when you need them.

Air Drying:

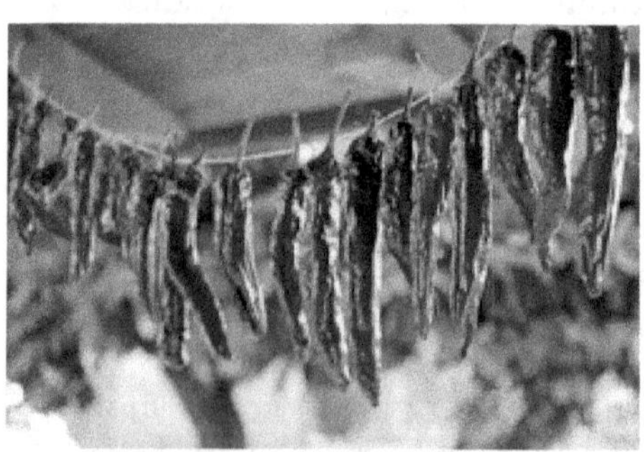

Many foods, such as hot peppers, can be strung together and simply hung, in an out of the way location, possibly on a beam or under a shelf to air dry, over time.

And, once they have dried, whenever you need a couple of hot peppers for cooking, or just a snack, simply pull one or two from the string and use them in your cooking, as they are needed.

Peppers dried this way, will be good for up to 2-3 years.

Some Drying Tips;

Typically, you should remove the seed from grapes, figs, dates and other such fruits before drying them.

When drying herbs and spices, remove the stems before drying and when the drying process is finished, store them in sealed containers to maintain their unique fragrance and flavors.

Remember that dried fruits will have a higher sugar content by weight than their undried counterpart.

Remember that properly dried meats, although they are still a great Protein and nutritional food source, will be tough and chewy and high in Salt when being consumed.

How to Build a Compost Pile

OK, so what is a Compost Pile, anyway?

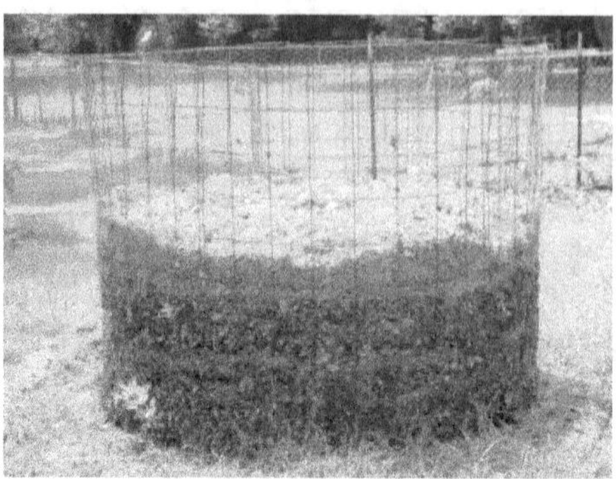

For those of you that might not be into gardening, a compost pit is a specially designed but at the same time, a simple place that you can use to place your biodegradables to rot.

Your excess food, plant trimmings and other debris is collected in this one spot to accelerate their degradation, or "rotting" into a state that it can be re-used.

The Compost is just an organic material made from wasted vegetable and other matter that has been allowed to rot to the point that it can be used as a fertilizer or soil additive to provide the basic nutrients for your next crops.

How to build your Compost Pile

This is one of my favorite and easiest ways to make a compost pile and below is a simplified instruction list to make your own pit.

1- First, you should **build a fenced area** about 6-feet by 6-feet and around 5-feet high.

Chicken wire or wire fencing works well for this. Simply roll it into a circle and connect the ends together.

The floor of your Compost heap must be **bare earth** in order to allow for the bugs that exist in the ground to access the compost waste.

2- To get your compost "working" initially, you should **place your vegetable and food waste in a layer** until it is about 6-inches in depth.

3- Ideally you should place **a layer of Fish Manure or Seaweed Manure** over the food waste, in an even layer.

If these are not available, use **Animal manure** such as Cow manure which might be available on your farm or you can purchase it reasonably at most Home Garden stores.

This combination will start working within days as you will be able to tell when it start generating heat from the rotting process.

Your compost pile is then built in layers, over time until the working pile has filled the compost piles walls.

4- **Water the compost** every couple of weeks to keep it moist, but do not keep it too wet.

5- If you find that your garden site's soil is **Acidic then you can add a little Lime** to the pile to change the pH level.

6- You should also use a pitchfork and **punch holes into the pile** every few days to allow more air to get to the compost and make it work faster.

7- **Cover your working compost pile** with something that will help keep the heat in the working compost and keep most of the rain out. Use pieces of old carpets or rugs, or an old plastic tarp that you have punched a lot of holes into which will allow the compost to breath and continue working on its own.

8- You should **climb into the compost pit and tread on the compost heap** once a week to pack the rotting materials down as it works the materials into fertilizer over time.

9- A typical compost pile **will take about a year** before the rotted material is ready for use on your garden, so like most people, you might want to eventually have two compost piles working.

Gardeners quickly find that the rich materials from a compost heap, once it is spread over the garden spot and tilled into the soil will really kick up the size and flavors of your garden crop.

Raising Livestock – Urban CHICKENS

Fresh Eggs year round, great tender chicken meat whenever you want and all of this, so cheap that it is embarrassing? It just sounds too good to be true, right?

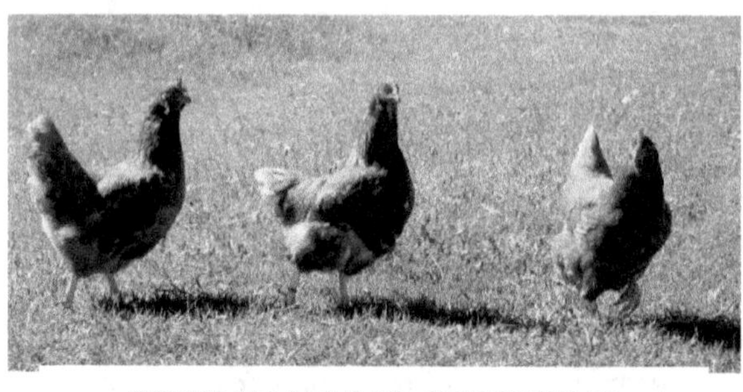

FREE RANGING CHICKENS

Well, owning and caring for your own Urban Chickens is something that many people can do at a relatively low investment and in a surprisingly small space.

I will not get into how to raise chickens on the scale of a farmer who has a family that eats and even sells large amounts of eggs and chickens for meat.

Rather, I well describe how you can get started, with just a few chickens and product a small but steady crop of eggs and occasionally even eat one of your chickens.

If you end up wanting to expand tour brood after a few months, then you can do so, but if you decide that there are better ways to spend your time then you will not have lost much money or time learning this lesson in survival farming.

There are a number of questions that you will have to ask yourself, if you do decide to raise chickens in large quantities. But if you just want to start out by producing enough fresh eggs for yourself and your family, then it can be a relatively easy task.

Chickens take Time

Raising Chickens requires a certain level of time commitment. To properly care for your birds you should probably count on spending from 30 minutes to an hour in the morning and the same amount of time in the evenings, every day.

That amount of time will be necessary for; feeding and watering your chickens, collecting Eggs, cleaning nests, inspecting your chicken coop and fenced lot for damage. And most importantly you need to constantly be on the lookout for signs of varmints that like to eat chickens.

Learn the local Law

You may be surprised to find that there are many town and cities that allow a homeowner to keep a few chickens for personal use as long as you follow their requirements.

Some locations do not allow property owners to raise any type of livestock, while others may allow a certain number of some animals, such a chickens.

But, at the same time, they may restrict such things as; the number of chickens allowed, whether there can be roosters or just hens, specifically how close they can be to neighbor's homes, etcetera.

Building a Chicken Coop

Keep in mind that Chickens have no natural defenses so predator animals such as foxes, dogs, raccoons and others need to be kept out of your birds home.

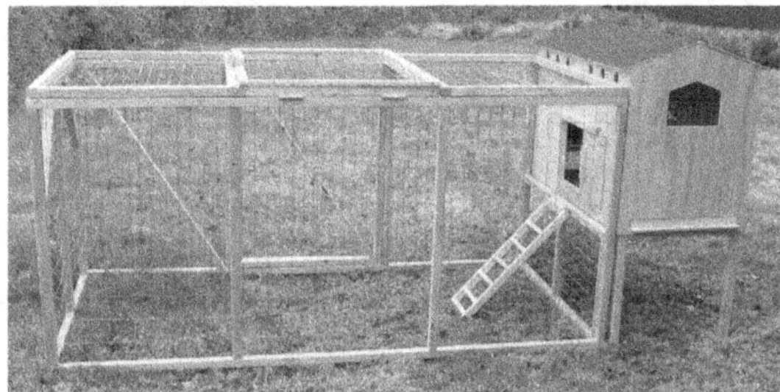

So you will need to build or purchase a Chicken Coop for the protection of your birds.

Whether you have a fancy chicken coop built, or if you just assemble your own out of whatever materials you might have or find (similar to the one shown below), remember that typically a coop should provide around two square feet of floor space for each chicken you own.

Free Range chickens that are allowed to roam a large area of open ground would require a little less coop space, but they do require a large range area, so try to keep to this 2 square feet guideline.

Basically, a chicken coop is just a simple shed with shelves installed for the birds to nest and sleep.

It is recommended that the shelves be made of wire, usually with ¼-inch square openings so that the manure drops to the floor for easy cleaning.

Regardless of what you use, all manure should be scraped from shelves, nests, and the floor of the coop regularly and not be allowed to build up. This manure is perfect for the growth of diseases and bacteria's.

Donald W Bobbitt

If you add a small area about the same size as the shed onto the front of the shed, made of chicken wire (and over 6-feet high), then you will have a nice space for the chickens to be range and feed on insects and to just walk about.

But, keep in mind that the larger the lot, the more opportunities there are for those Varmints to get in and eat your chickens or even for your chickens to find a hole and escape.

If you have a much larger area for you chickens to pasture at times during the day, your chickens will get more protein and other minerals and they will produce eggs with brown shells and bright orange yolks.

Again though, the fenced area and the shed combination should be built strong and tall enough to keep predators out of the chicken coop.

Buying Chickens for egg production

If it were me, I would start with raising chickens just for the egg production and if I wanted to raise them for the meat, I could modify my plans later.

There are a number of breeds of chicken that are either better for their meat or for their eggs. The novice should probably contact a local hatchery or an online one who ships young chicks and get their suggestions on which kind their first chickens should be.

Rhode Island Reds and **Leghorns** are probably the two most popular egg-laying breeds available. They are hearty breeds that provide a relatively large number of eggs. And, they can start producing eggs when they are 3-6 months old.

Build a simple Brooder

If you purchase chicks then you will need to build a simple brooder.

Depending on the number of chicks you get, a brooder can be just a shoebox, a wooden box or whatever you have that keeps the young chicks contained.

Place the brooder in your garage, basement or some other warm space, line the bottom with old newspapers and put your young chicks into the brooder.

Place a lamp over the brooder and try to keep the temperature at around 90F the first week, dropping the temperature by five degrees a week until you reach 80F, as a rule of thumb.

84

Keep an eye on your chicks, one tip is if they are cold they will huddle together and if they are hot they will stay away from each other.

Change the paper liner out every 2-3 days feed them properly and they will "feather out" or grow actual feathers in about six weeks.

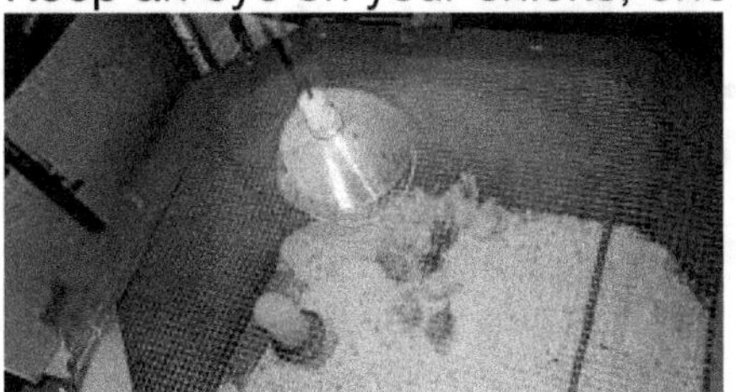

BROODER for Young Chicks

Feeding Chickens

New chicks should be fed a medicated starter mix that is especially designed for young birds and also includes certain needed medications.

They should be kept on this special feed until the birds have feathered-out. Then they can be moved to the actual coop and fed regular chicken feed.

Chickens also need water but they are not very smart birds so be aware if you use a bowl or some other device other than a **Chick Waterer**, you are going to lose some of your chicks.

They will drown in the water, turn the bowl over, or get cold from being wet. **Chick Waterers** and **Adult Bird Waterers** can be purchased from local hatcheries or just look for one you can purchase nearby on the web.

There are special feeds for egg bearing chickens and they should be either a layer pellet or a layer mash brand that will provide the full range of nutrients they need for producing strong healthy eggs.

Chickens that are not allowed to range or pasture will need to be fed a mixture that includes a grit that is stored in their craw and helps them digest their food.

Chicken Health

Chickens are generally healthy if they are cared for properly. But at times you may walk into your coop and find a dead bird, or maybe one that is acting strangely.

You will rarely know what makes your chicken die or appear ill, but it is always a good idea to isolate the ill ones from the others and just kill it.

Donald W Bobbitt

Once a chicken begins to show signs of being ill, it is seriously ill and the easiest thing to do is just destroy the bird. And, of courses, do not eat the meat of sick chickens; discard them immediately.

Your Chickens and Your Health

With all of this in mind, you will find that you can be raising chickens for eggs is a pretty simple process that has great and healthy returns for a small amount of work as well as a minimal investment.

Once you research the basics of raising chickens, you can end up with not only a steady supply of fresh eggs year round, but you can also have the occasional fresh, chicken for your table.

And, of course, your eggs and chickens will not be raised under cruel conditions nor will they have been fed the hormones, antibiotics and other drugs that our FDA allows the commercial growers to use.

Egg Production

Just a few chickens will produce enough eggs for you and your family, year round even though their output will often vary with the seasons.

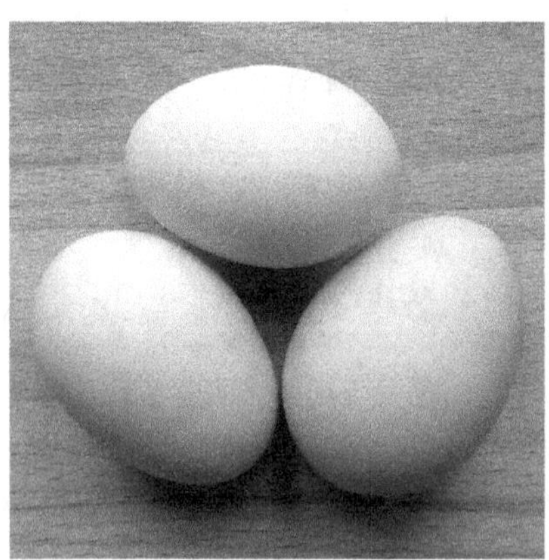

Your typical healthy egg producing chicken will produce for 4-6 years and can actually live for up to ten years, with their egg production dropping off after the second year.

At this point you need to decide if you are going to eat your older chickens or just get rid of them, especially if you have formed and attachment with some of them.

I, personally love to eat chicken, pretty much any way you what to prepare them; fried, baked, broiled and especially cooked in a crockpot with some veggies.

But, the beginner needs to prepare themselves for their first chicken kill. The killing is easy, but if you are going to eat the chicken, getting rid of those feathers can be a real task.

Look up the right procedures for killing and cleaning a chicken before you start on this task.

In the summer you can expect your young and well fed chickens to produce, on average, 5-6 eggs a week, each, with the older ones producing less.

This number will drop in the winter when the days are shorter. Some people place a light, on a timer, to generate more light making the chickens think it is still summer.

As to any extra eggs, you can always offer them to your neighbors, friends or relatives as a treat. Always wash the fresh eggs and assure that they do not have any manure dark spots on them as this will really turn off your uneducated friends.

And, of course, you can always take these extra eggs to your local farmers market and sell them there,

Bad things for Chickens

When you feed your chickens you do not want to give them foods that might affect your eggs and there are some specific foods that you should avoid feeding to your chickens altogether.

Do not feed your chickens foods that include strong flavors like Onions, Garlic and Leeks as these can change the flavor of your eggs. Another concern is that Green Potatoes can be toxic to chickens.

Keep your chickens away from certain **plants that are poisonous to chickens**, such as: Avocado, Azalea, Columbine, Goldenrod and Trumpet Vine to name a few.

Chickens will eat almost anything they find while ranging, and some debris will damage their digestive systems, such as; Styrofoam, metals, paper and pieces of string.

Raising Livestock –URBAN PIGS

Many people do not realize that they can raise an Urban Pig or two on their property, often even in the city, with very little effort or expense.

 Of course, before you get too excited about having your own supply of pork, you need to check the local laws on raising pigs and also make sure you are aware of any restrictions or special requirements.

Once you are satisfied that the legal restrictions are on your side you can then get into the process of preparation for raising your own pigs at home.

First of all, few urban farmers will want to even attempt to raise a full sized pig breed such as a Berkshire or Tamworth. These breeds

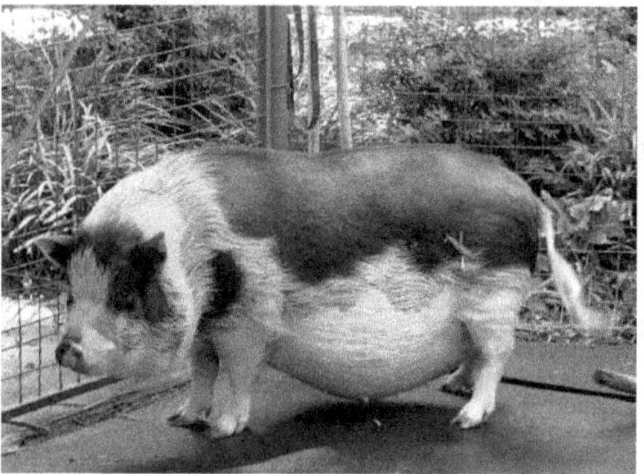

grow very large, in the hundreds of pounds each but they require a large amount of living space and are voracious eaters.

Most urban farmers will raise just one or two breeder pigs that are small and easily controlled such as what are often called "Weiner Pigs".

A couple of popular examples are the **Kunekune** and **Pot-Bellied Pig** breeds. These smaller pigs require very little space and you can set up a reasonable space in your backyard with just the following materials:

- A **Dog House** - for protection of one Pig from the weather or a simple 4-foot by 4-foot shelter can suffice.
- A **Water Trough** – this can be as simple as a few wooden planks nailed together.
- A **Feeding Trough** – this should be made of metal for ease of cleaning.
- A **Water Source** and carry container,
- **Pig Feed** and a dry space out of the weather for storage,
- **Straw for bedding** - to keep the Pig Pen dry and clean and most importantly of all, this will require regular changing.

- A good **Electric Fence** - set up several rings of electric fence designed to contain your Pig from getting loose. A loose Pig can quickly destroy other plants in your Back Yard.

Once you find a breeder to purchase your Pig from, make sure that if it is a male, it has been castrated and the wound has healed before you pick it up.

Feeding your Pig:

These Weiner Pigs will consume between 0.5 and 1.5 pounds of food a day, 0.5-lbs. when young and small and up to 1.5-lbs.a day when they are adults.

Most people will depend on feed pellets as the basic feed for their pigs but you can supplement their feed with food scraps to cut your costs a little. If you had access to a forest area, you could take these little pigs out for a walk occasionally and let them forage to their hearts content, but remember they can tear a yard up if you let them loose so keep them penned up at all times.

Some people will even make friends with their local grocer and offer to take their bad (not rotten, but bad) vegetables off of their hands. Pigs will wolf these vegetables down as quickly as they will their packaged feeds.

One note though, even though they will eat and eat, do not overfeed your Pig as it can become sick and even die under certain circumstances. Keep their food limited to what is recommended for a healthy Pig.

Housing Your Pig

As has been mentioned, you can start with a simple plastic Dog House for one Pig, or you can build a simple shelter from planks cover it with a tin or plastic roof. But, be sure to raise the floor above the ground level.

Pigs are not neat animals, and a pigpen with a raised floor can be easily hosed out regularly and fresh straw added on the floor to keep the smell down and keep the pig dry and healthy.

Your Pigs Health

First of all, make sure that when you purchase your small Pig that it has had shots for Worms. Also, remember that you need have them treated for Worms every 4-6 months.

Over time you may have problems with other diseases common to pigs, but a pig that is well fed, and kept in a dry and airy living area will not be nearly as susceptible to parasites and diseases as others that are not managed as well.

It is a good idea when making your little pig pen area to design it so that it can be easily moved to a different location in your yard every few months to help avoid the development of parasites that can attack your pig.

Remember that a healthy pig is a hungry and active pig, while a sick pig is a lethargic one that isn't eating well. If you notice these symptoms, check with your breeder or other knowledgeable source on what to do next.

Slaughter Time

At some point, your pig will have grown to the point that you are ready to have it slaughtered and the meat cut up for you. Again, check with the breeder that you originally purchased your Pig from and he will be able to tell you of someone who can take care of this chore for you.

In my youth, when I lived in the country, I helped family, and friends, kill and "Put Up" a lot of pigs.

It's an art in itself and before you attempt to do this yourself, I recommend that you find someone skilled at this task and ask them to let you help a few times just to learn the tricks of the trade.

You can learn the process and not lose very much of the edible meat, or you can just jump in with a knife and end up with a lot of waste if you have never done this before.

I remember my grandparents used to brag that, **"When we Killed a Hog we put up everything but the Squeal!"**

Homemade Laundry Detergent

When you go to the supermarket and pick up a container of laundry detergent you can go into sticker shock. As you may already know, a good laundry detergent is a very expensive commodity for the average homeowner.

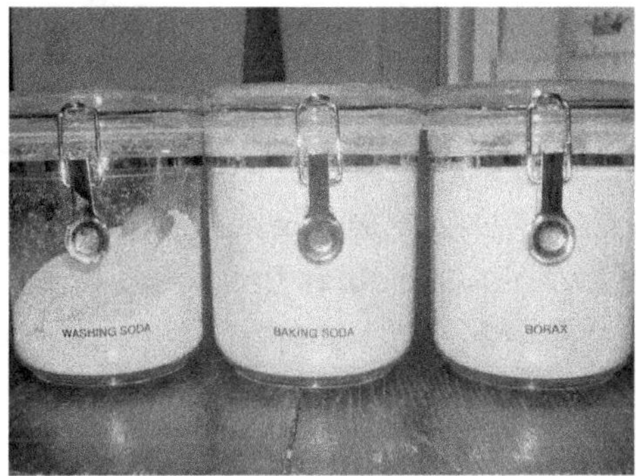

But, many people do not realize that they can make a good, high quality laundry detergent for themselves, and at a very low cost.

Making such simple items as your own laundry detergent, for your personal home use is not just better for the environment and your family budget.

When you make your own, you are also leaving out the artificial scents and toxic chemicals used by commercial laundry detergent manufacturers.

How to Make a Homemade Laundry Detergent

There are many simple formulas available for use in making very good laundry detergents that you can start using right now.

In reality, if you are a good shopper, you can accumulate the ingredients for a good laundry detergent that will wash up to 100 loads of clothes for less than $2.00.

Simple Laundry detergent recipe;

First, you must combine; 6-cups of **Naptha Soap** (or **Zote Soap**), grated, with 3 cups of **Mule Team Borax** along with the same amount of **Arm and Hammer Washing Soda**.

To this mixture, add 8-10 drops of **Lavender Essential Oil**, for its fresh and natural Lavender scent. Remember, you can experiment with other Essential Oils for the one that gives you the aroma you like the best.

Mix the ingredients together well and then place it in a covered container for at least 24-hours for the ingredients to blend together well.

To use this great homemade laundry detergent, just add two tablespoons of the mixture to a normal load of wash.

Be aware that this homemade detergent will inherently have fewer suds than the commercial brands but otherwise it will still keep your clothes as clean as the commercial brands.

Again, remember that if you want to change the scent of your clean clothes, you can just change the essential oil you used to another one with an aroma you might prefer or you can even mix several Essential Oils together to eventually get whatever aroma you personally prefer.

NOTE: For safety's sake, keep your homemade detergent covered and away from children, just as you would any other detergent or household cleanser.

Making Your Own SOAPS

Soap is such a simple everyday thing that we all use but, at the same time, we know very little about soaps and how they are made.

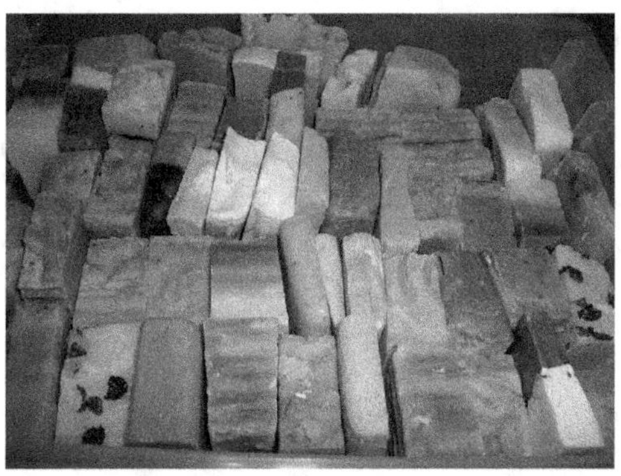

As we all know, soaps can be more than a cleanser for the body, but if they are made with the appropriate ingredients, they can moisturize and even help protect the skin.

The problem for some of us is the fact that many of the commercial soaps are not soaps at all but contain detergents and other chemicals that can not only pollute the environment, some can even have damaging effects on your skin.

So, it is no surprise that many Survivalists will end up making their own **Homemade Soaps** or at least purchasing homemade soaps that they can trust.

SOAP MAKING Processes

Soap-making itself is a relatively simple process, and when you learn the few special tricks to the trade, you can make a great environmentally friendly and healthy soap of your own.

You will quickly find that it will not only be cheaper to make your own soap but your personalized soap can have a fragrance that suits your personal taste while at the same time it will be one that will moisturize your skin, using natural and safe ingredients.

If you are interested in making your own soaps, there are several procedures that you can use depending on whether you just want to make small amounts of soap for your personal use or if you want to share some with friends or even if you want to sell it at craft stores and shows to make a few bucks.

There are a number or procedures that you can follow for making homemade soaps, such as Quick-Cure Soaps, Cold-Process Soaps and Hot-Process Soaps. Each of these procedures has advantages and disadvantages for the individual Survivalist who is interested in making his own soaps.

Castille or Olive Oil Soap

This **Cold-Process Soap** has been made for hundreds of years and has always been popular for being a mild, Skin Moisturizer soap that produces a lot of lather.

Before you start making this soap, make sure that you have the appropriate tools on hand especially your gloves and goggles for protection.

And, to be a successful soap maker, you had better be good at measuring your ingredients precisely, or your soap will fail to come out right.

Simplified Recipe for this popular soap:
1. Place 9-oz. of distilled water into your clean dry stainless steel pan.
2. Add precisely 3.49 oz. of Red Devil Lye to the water, and mix together well with a wooden spoon.
3. Allow the mixture to sit and it will heat itself. Monitor the temperature and when the temp peaks and then when it drops just below 120F, (but make sure it stays at a temperature of at least 100F) continue the process.
4. While the Lye mixture is working, mix; 8-ox of Olive Oil, 8-oz. of Coconut Oil and 8-oz. of rendered tallow together, over a medium heat, slowly and once everything is melted and blended, drop the temperature of this mixture to between 100F and 120F.
5. Making sure that the Lye mixture and the Oil mixture are both at the same temperature, (between 100F and 120F) add the Oils mixture to the Lye mixture.
6. TRACING – Stir the combined mixtures for about 15-minutes, until it reaches the consistency of a pudding. Once tracing is reached, slowly pour the mixture into a mold or shallow tray or plastic bin and set it aside for 2-3 days to set up properly.
7. Inspect the soap for pockets of Lye, as these can be dangerous to you if you get the lye on your skin when handling the soap block or bars.
8. Allow the large block of soap to sit for another day or so before cutting it into bars.
9. Finally, wrap the soap bars in rags and allow them to sit in a cool dry place for at least two weeks before use.

Potential Problems: There are a number of problems that can occur with a homemade soap process. A typical one is that streaks occur in the soap. Streaks are a sign of too much Lye or of poor mixing, The Lye must be pure, the water must be distilled and the measurements must be precise or the soap may not set up.

Other great Soap Recipes

There are many other great recipes for homemade soaps that are easy to find on the web and in health food stores.

The Fats used in Soaps:

There are a number of common fats that are popularly used in Soap recipes, here are some of the different affects these fats may have on your Homemade Soap:

Beef Fat – makes a soap that is soft and slippery

Coconut Oil - makes a soap with a nice lather.

Lard – makes a mild soap.

Olive Oil – makes a mild soap that may be brittle and break easily.

Palm Oil – makes a soap with lots of bubbles.

Tallow – makes a good soap with bubbles.

Popular Additives for Cold Process Soaps

There are a number of popular additives that you can use in your homemade soaps and here below are a few.

If you want to try these and other Essential Oils in your soaps for either their health properties or just for their pleasing aroma, it only takes a couple of drops of the oil in your formula.

Additive	Properties
Coconut Oil	Makes Good Lather, Moisturizer, anti-inflammatory, good for skin conditions.
Coffee, ground	Deodorizer
Hempseed Oil	Anti-Oxidant, healing properties
Lavender Oil	Nice Flowery scent
Olive Oil	Moisturizer, seals moisture into skin, is a soap hardener.
Shea Butter	Moisturizer, Emollient, fights skin damage

TOOTHPASTE – Make your own

Toothpaste is actually a simple product anyone can make themselves.

Toxins in Your Toothpaste?

Most commercial toothpastes contain fluoride among other toxic ingredients you can read about on the web.

If you read the label on most toothpaste's, especially the ones that contain fluorides, you will see FDA required warnings about some of the ingredients.

Most commercial toothpastes will also contain sodium lauryl sulfate, which is often added as a preservative that will dry your mouth and can cause canker sores.

Many commercial toothpastes are sweetened with saccharin, which has a spotted history of being known as a cancer-causing agent that we are all familiar with.

Make your own simple Toothpaste

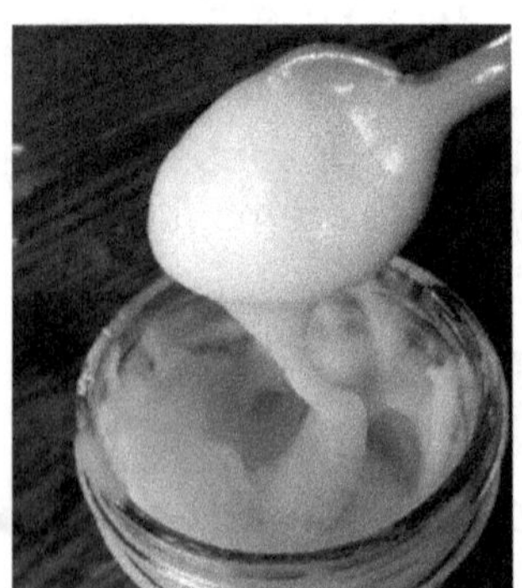

When you get down to it, the available products are just simple and safe, flavored pastes that aren't very different from each other.

Homemade Toothpaste, like its commercial counterparts, are so simple the process for making your own is an easy thing for you to try.

Below is a simple recipe for you to make your own toothpaste get the same results as the commercial versions and you can modify the flavors to suit your personal tastes.

Common Ingredients for Homemade Toothpastes:

Teeth Cleaning Powders- Popular powders that you can use are; **Baking Soda, Bentonite Clay Powder, Sage Powder** and **Mint Powder** to name a few of the more popular ones.

Baking Soda is a good whitener and deodorizer.

Bentonite Clay powder is a good yet mild abrasive.

Dried Sage, ground into a powder is a natural tooth whitener and adding ground up Dried Mint you'll get a great flavoring to offset the rough flavor of the Sage.

Adding Essential Oils to your toothpaste –

There are several popular Essential Oils to use in toothpaste that you can use.

- **Coconut Oil** is not only flavorful but it is a natural antibacterial that kills germs and reduces tooth plaque.
- **Olive Oil** can be used to save money but you do not get the same health benefits as with Coconut Oil.
- **Tea Tree Oil** is a great germ killer and is good for the teeth and gums overall.
- You can also add small amounts of other natural ingredients such as; **Mint Oil** freshens the breath and kills germs, **Cinnamon powder** or small amounts of ground **Cloves** can be added to treat a sore mouth, but only use a little as using both can irritate sore gums.

Basic Toothpaste Recipe:

The recipe below is a good one for the first-time toothpaste maker.

1. Place 1-tablespoon of Coconut oil into a sterile bowl
2. Add 5-7 drops of Mint Oil to the bowl (or use Cinnamon Oil, Clove or a combination of the two if you like a spicy toothpaste)
3. Add ½ teaspoon of Sea Salt to the bowl
4. Add Baking Soda to the bowl, slowly, while blending until you have a thick paste.
5. Mix the ingredients together well and then place it in a small, sterile sealable container

To use, just open the container, dip your toothbrush into the paste and brush your teeth with your own great tasting and healthy toothpaste. And, once you have made your own toothpaste, you can experiment with flavors of Oils and powders to customize your toothpaste to your personal needs and then make your toothpaste in larger quantities.

NOTE: Most homemade toothpaste formulas do not foam like the store bought versions, so you will often need to remix the paste to keep it at the right consistency.

LIFESTYLE Tips and Tools

Here is a collection of miscellaneous tips and tools that they do not teach you in school but can prove to be very useful for a Survivalist.

Most are things that you can do yourself rather than count on large corporations for their products.

And, some of these are just simple knowledge that you can use in your every day life that if you apply them, you will be taking one more step towards becoming a more independent individual.

For want of a way to present these little jewels of wisdom, that are presented alphabetically.

<u>Aftershave Lotion, Make your own</u>

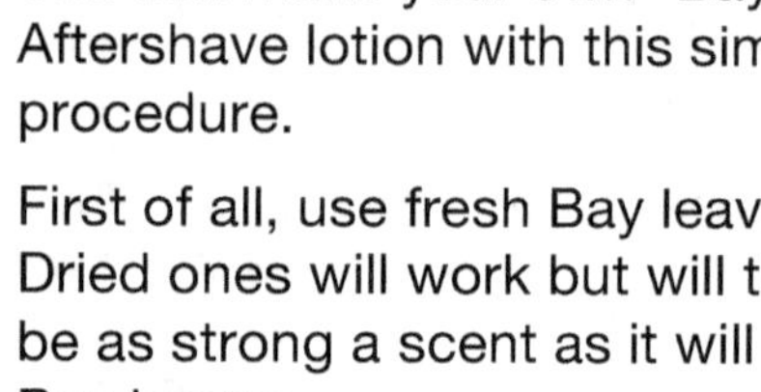

You can make your own "Bay Rum" Aftershave lotion with this simple procedure.

First of all, use fresh Bay leaves if possible. Dried ones will work but will the results not be as strong a scent as it will be with fresh Bay leaves.

Fill a large jar with Bay leaves and add:

2-tbs of ground Allspice,

1-tsp of whole Cloves, with

2-tbs of ground Ginger.

Fill the jar one-third of the way with water and then fill the rest of the way with a low-cost Rum, making sure that the liquid covers the other ingredients by an inch or more.

Seal the jar and set it aside in a warm place for four to five weeks making sure to shake the jar well once or twice each week. Once the mixture has aged, strain the liquid into another sealable jar and you will have your herbal liquid astringent that can be used as a great aftershave lotion.

You can add a few drops of Oil of Bay to the mixture for an even stronger and longer lasting scent.

Aging Beef

Aging Beef for a certain period of time can not only provide it with a longer life before you need to use it but aging can also improve the flavors of the meat. Beef can be either Dry Aged or Wet Aged.

Dry Aged beef is a very expensive process and entails hanging beef in places with well-controlled temperatures for a specific period of time, generally from 15-28 days.

Typically, there is a significant loss of weight due to lost moisture. Dry Aged Beef is usually sold in high end Steak Houses.

Wet Aging Beef takes only a few days and is the process of taking a cut of beef and vacuum sealing the cut in a plastic bag. Wet aging allows for almost no moisture lass and is by far the predominant method of aging beef and certain other meats in the US.

Aging Fruits and Vegetables

Almost all Fruits and Vegetables generate ethylene gases as they age. These gases, if trapped around the fruit, will cause the fruit or vegetable itself to age or ripen much sooner than when it is stored or displayed in the open air.

Some of the ones that generate the highest levels of ethylene are; Apricots, Avocados, Bananas, Cantalopes, Melons, Kiwis, Mangoes, Peaches, Pears Plums and Tomatoes.

And, of course, there are certain fruits and vegetables that are very susceptible to ethylene gases and will grow spots, and become soft relatively fast are: Apples, Asparagus, Broccoli, Carrots, Cucumbers, Eggplant, Green Beans, Greens, Potatoes, Summer Squash and Watermelons.

One tip though, if you purchase certain of these fresh foods that are not quite ripe enough for you, place them in a paper bag for a day or so, and their own gases will accelerate their ripening.

You should carefully check your packaged fresh foods for prematurely aged items in the package. Often you will find rotted fruits that are in sealed packages and these contained gases often cause this problem with the more mature pieces.

Donald W Bobbitt

Canning and Pickling, a food storage tool

The Canning and Pickling of excess crops is a great way to store foods for later use. If it is done properly, many canned foods can last for up to ten years or more. Before they go bad.

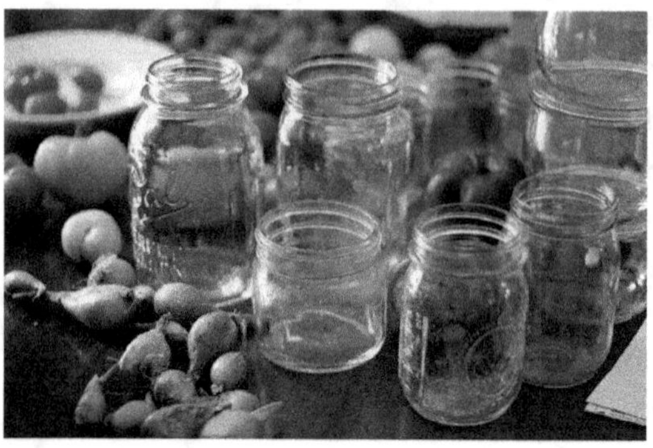

Pickling is simply the process of covering a food with an acidic or sugar-rich liquid, placing it into a sealable container and over time, through fermentation, the acids or sugars prevent bacteria from attacking the food in the container.

The liquids and spices used in the pickling process drop the pH level of the food to a level below 4.6, which is low enough to prevent the growth of most bacteria's.

Vinegar is the preferred liquid used for pickling and imparts a spicy and tart flavor to the pickled foods.

Certain Herbs and Spices such as Cinnamon, Cloves Garlic, Mustard seeds and Onion are often added not only for their flavor, but also for their anti-microbial properties. Salt also aids the pickling process.

Canning is a more complex process used for preparing foods for storage. Once, foods were prepared and actually stored in unlined tin cans. These cans would leech lead into the foods and made the foods toxic to the people who consumed the foods.

 A few decades ago, all cans were lines with plastics, which prevented this leeching of lead and other metals into the canned foods.

The problem now is that most canned foods, packaged in metal cans, are line with BPA plastics, which have been found to cause certain cancers.

Today, some canned foods are packaged in glass jars designed specifically for the canning process. Although more expensive to use than metal cans, disposable glass canning jars are used by many commercial food producers for certain foods.

Canning foods with a reusable jar design are the most popular methods of canning used by the small farmer.

The Canning Process:

The food is prepared to a specific recipe, and then it is placed into sterilized canning jars. The jars are "sealed" use metal lids that have separate tops that seal the jar.

The jars are essentially scalded in boiling water for a period of time, which removes the bacteria in the food itself. Then the jars are removed from the water and allowed to cool. As the mixture in the jar cools it contracts and the suction pulls the jar seal closed.

Canning vegetables and other foods, requires that the foods be prepared properly to the appropriate recipe for the canning process to be a success.

Improperly canned foods will spoil in the jars and eventually the pressure from the growing bacteria can cause the jars to explode, or to turn bad.

Cooking Oils, Rancid

If they are not stored properly your cooking oils can often go bad and turn rancid over time after they are opened.

Because of their anti-bacterial properties, you should consider placing a few twigs of your favorite Herb into the bottle of Oil.

For instance, by placing a twig or two of Rosemary into your opened bottles of cooking oils, such as Olive Oil, you can help keep the oil from going rancid for a longer period of time.

In fact, the oils useful life can be extended for up to three months longer by adding such anti-bacterial Herbs.

As an added consequence, the oils from the Rosemary will leech into the Olive Oil and impart that great rosemary flavor that so many people love to the dishes you prepare with the oil.

Fabric Softener, Homemade

Fabric Softeners are popular wherever the public water supply is determined to be "hard". But, rather than using the commercial solutions, making a homemade fabric softener is actually quite simple.

You can make a simple fabric softener by mixing ¼-cup of Vinegar with a few drops of your favorite scented essential oil. Add this mixture to the washing machine during the rinse cycle and the combination of vinegar and oil will give your clothes a soft feel and a fresh smell.

Another recipe for making a fabric softener is to mix one cup of baking soda with one cup of vinegar. Blend the mixture together well and add it your washing machine during the rinse cycle.

Freezing Foods, How to

If you want to use your freezer efficiently, you need to understand how to properly freeze the foods that you want to keep there.

Few people understand that those very cold aisles in the supermarket with all of those glass doors displaying such a wide variety of frozen foods can be a goldmine for the average consumer.

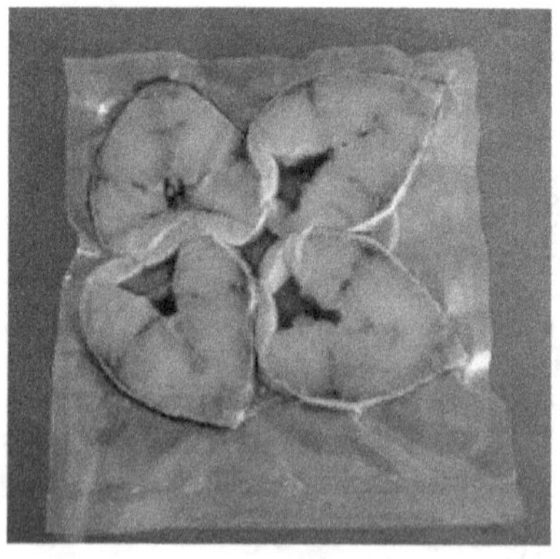

One advantage of using fresh frozen foods versus canned is the fact that they have not been cooked and thus they have not lost any of their vitamins and minerals to the high temperatures often used to cook their canned counterparts.

You may not know that most agri-business companies actually pick the fruits and vegetables that you see in those froze plastic bags and, within a couple of hours of harvesting, they clean, process and freeze the food. Now that's fresh.

You will find that properly frozen foods can save you a lot of money whether you purchase what is in the supermarket or if you freeze it yourself.

Improperly frozen foods can suffer from "frostbite" or freezer burn, dry out and lose much of their fresh flavor.

Most fresh foods, especially fruits and vegetables freeze better if it is cut up into pieces and you will often see commercially frozen foods that are pre-cut.

Your leftovers are best if they are placed into a freezer bag or other airtight container and have the excess air removed before they are freezing. It's that extra air that allows space for the frozen food to degrade in the freezer.

On the other hand take care with Rice and Pasta dishes. They will freeze better and last longer if they are actually covered with the sauces they were prepared in, before they are frozen.

Always take care when attempting to freeze liquids, as they will require a small amount of air at the top of the container to allow for the expansion of the liquid when it freezes.

Honey and Infants, a Warning!

In addition to its fantastic taste, Honey is so good for so many things that you would think it was harmless.

But you should **never give honey to an infant under 12-months old**. Honey can be poisonous to infants because it grows spores known as botulinum; which can, under certain conditions, lead to food poisoning or even paralysis in an infant.

Once a child has grown to be over 12- months old, its intestines (and the intestinal bacteria) are strong enough to destroy these particular spores.

Household Cleanser, Make your own

There are a lot of household cleansers on the market today, but people are not aware that it is actually very easy to make one of your own that is cheaper than the store bought versions and is eco-friendly because it does not contain the dangerous chemicals often found in many commercial versions.

RECIPE: Mix together; ¼ cup of Vinegar (or Vodka?) with 1-cup of distilled water and then add 10 to 20 drops of your favorite smelling Essential Oil.

Shake the mixture well and then place it in a spray bottle and use as necessary on your typical household dirt and stains. Be aware that the mixture's scent does not last for a long time so it is best to just make a small amount, as shown, at a time.

I recommend that you use the Vinegar, as opposed to the Vodka, and you will have a general household cleaner and disinfectant that you can use to wipe down your whole house.

How much Land does a Survivalist need

Many Survivalists will eventually end up asking themselves the question; Just how much land do I need to survive on, planting my own crops, heating my home with wood, and raising my own livestock?

Decades ago, when I lived in Central Virginia, I read an article in the popular magazine called Mother Earth News (MEN) about how much wooded land was needed for a family of four to heat their home and Cook their foods year round.

At that time, MEN recommended that, in the Central part of the Eastern USA, if a family of four had ten acres of wooded land, then they could heat their home and cook their foods using only the deadfall and cut wood from diseased trees. By doing this, they would never run out of wood on their property.

Of course, location is very important and in other areas of the country would have different requirements to survive. And, a survivalist or even a part-time survivalist would need more land than this or growing crops and raising their livestock but this is a good indication of just one land requirement.

For even more great information on farming and survival techniques, I suggest that you see the Mother Earth News website. I can tell you that they are an unbelievable source of information for a survivalist.

Raising Beef, land needed

If you want to raise livestock, I have seen it recommended that you plan on having at least one full acre of land to support every 1000 pounds of grazing cows. And, in reality, at times you will probably still need to supplement their feeding with hay and even cattle feeds.

Imported Fruits and Vegetables, watch out!

In case you didn't realize it, today, **over 60%** of the fresh fruits and vegetables sold and consumed in the US are from other countries.

In fact, as crazy as it sounds, much of what is grown in the US is shipped to other countries, mostly due to the high prices that US grown and raised foods demand overseas.

When I first found this out, I asked myself; is this a case of brilliant advertising on our part? Or, is it something else like maybe they want to eat better and safer foods, just like we do?

You might even ask yourself; "What are the production, feeding and cleaning standards of these other countries?"

And how do they regulate the chemicals used to improve their production volumes. Some countries do have health standards for foods produced there, but many do not.

In fact, we purchase much of our foreign produced foods from companies in other countries where even though the nation itself does not have adequate standards, our FDA will sign contracts with the companies to produce there to our standards.

Of course the FDA is notoriously short of Inspector staff that might actually inspect that these companies really do follow our standards.

MAPLE SYRUP Grades

Maple Syrup a natural and delicious food used mostly as a

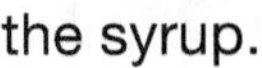

condiment on such food dishes as pancakes and waffles.

Its unique sweet flavor is so popular that nearly everyone loves to use it.

When you go out to purchase your own maple syrup you should be aware that the syrups themselves are graded for your convenience.

Maple Syrup is available in four grades that are based on the Color and Flavor of the syrup.

Below is a table that illustrates the differences in the grades.

Grade A Light	This mild flavored syrup is light in color and is harvested in the early Spring. It is normally used to make Maple Candies, Sugars and Maple Cream.
Grade A Medium	This stronger flavored syrup is harvested mid-season and is also used to make Maple Cream and Sugar. It is used as a table syrup and preferred on; Pancakes, Ice Cream and even on Oatmeal.
Grade A Dark	This very strong flavored syrup is harvested during the last month or so of the season and is typically used for cooking.
Grade B	This strong and dark syrup is harvested at the very end of the season and is used mostly for coking.

Mouthwash, Make your Own

Using a Mouthwash is something you can do that is both refreshing for your mouth and breath and that can, at the same time; kill germs in your mouth.

Commercial Mouthwash products often contain a number of strange ingredients such as what I see on the bottle label of my favorite. It lists the active ingredients as Eucalyptus (0.092%). Menthol (0.042%) Methyl Salicylates (0.06%) and Thymol (0.064%) that are all listed as being anti-gingivitis and anti-plaque additives.

The other inactive ingredients are; Water, Alcohol (21.6%), Sorbitol solution (?), flavor (?), Poloxamar 407 (?), Benzoic Acid, Sodium Saccharin, Sodium Benzoate, FD&C green 3.

I looked some of these up on the web and I threw the mouthwash in the trash. Fear will do that you a person.

Natural Mouthwash Recipe

RECIPE: Just combine ½-cup of distilled water with, ½ tsp.-Salt and 1-tsp.-Baking Soda.

Then add the Essential Oil, Tea Tree Oil (2-drops) that is an anti-bacterial, and (4-drops) Mint Oil, which has a great flavor and is also an anti-bacterial.

The recipe can be multiplied but remember, the Oils used, like so many Essential Oils will lose their potency and aroma after a couple of weeks.

You should place the homemade mouthwash in a sealable sterile jar and just make a small amount that will last you a week or two, like above, and the oils will not lose their strength from sitting too long.

MUM MOSQUITO Repellant

Although we humans love Mums for their beautiful blooms as well as the scent of the flowers, Mosquitos are repelled by their scent. So, a few strategically placed potted Mums can make your porch a more pleasant place to sit in the evening.

RECIPE: To make a natural mosquito repellant using Mums, do the following;

Chop a dozen or more Mum blossoms finely and place them into a small cotton bag. Soak the bag in 6-ounces of Olive Oil or Sunflower Oil, in a jar for at least two weeks.

Once fermented, filter the liquid from the mash and place the liquid into a sealable amber jar.

Use it by rubbing a drop or two onto pulse points of the body to ward off mosquitos. The liquid can be kept for a month or so or until it becomes rancid smelling.

SMOKED MEATS

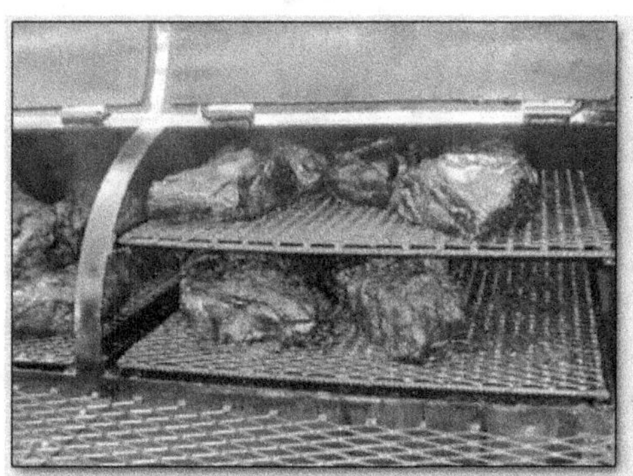

Almost any meat can be smoked to cure it, from Fish to Beef, Pork and Wild Game such as Deer, Elk, Boar, and others.

The trick to smoking meats is to realize that this process is great for imparting great wood and even herbal flavors to meats, but should not be considered a way to process and store meats for long period s of time.

The more popular woods to use when smoking meats are the aromatic ones such as, **Apple, Hickory, Elm, Mesquite, Cherry**, and **Sassafras**. But you may find people using pretty much any wood that will burn slowly and has a nice scent when you smell the wood that can be imparted to the meats.

On the other hand you need to avoid certain woods like Pine; which has a high pine tar content as this will coat the meat and leave a bad flavor.

Meat Temperatures

When handling, storing or preparing meats you need to know the **proper temperatures** for handling and processing your meats effectively and safely:

- **32F or lower** – Properly sealed meats can be frozen for long periods of time, even for several months.
- **40F or lower** – Meat can be stored safely at this temperature, but only for short periods of time.
- **40F-140F** – Meats kept at these temperatures are highly susceptible to Bacteria growth and should be consumed in a couple of days.
- **160F of higher** – Cooked meats are considered to be safe for consumption for a longer period of time typically 3-4 days.
- **190F - 220F** – Smoked meats should be cooked in this temperature range for safe consumption.
- **275F - 300F** – Barbecue and Slow Cook meats at this temperature.

SHAMPOO, Make your Own

People spend a lot of money on Shampoos for many different reasons. In fact, every drugstore and supermarket will have several shelves filled with every imaginable variety of cents and oils and other chemicals.

If you want a simple shampoo that cleans your hear and leaves it healthy, you might want to try making your own.

There are so many recipes for making a shampoo that I decided to list this one because of its simplicity. If you use it and it works, you can customize it to your own tastes.

Natural Homemade Shampoo Recipe:

Ingredients:

- ¼-cup Coconut Milk
- 1/3=cup Liquid Castille Soap
- 15-20 drops of your favorite Essential Oil (Lavender, Orange, Peppermint, and other fragrant Oils that you might like the scent of will work well, separately or in combinations).

Combine the ingredients together well and place the mixture in an old sterilized, shampoo bottle or a jar with a sealable top.

If you have dry hair, you can add ½-tsp. of Olive Oil to the mixture to get a more luxurious feeling to your hair.

The mixture will last up to a month before the Oils lose their strength, so only make enough to use for a couple of weeks at a time.

VENISON JERKY SAUSAGES – Simple Recipe

Making Sausages is a great way to use up those small pieces of meat you have left over when you kill your livestock or even wild game. They are easy to make and can be dried or cooked for a longer storage time

Venison Jerky Sausages

These sausages are not really, true "Dried Jerky", but they do taste great and are easy to make.

First of all, as most outdoorsmen know, Venison has very little fat content and can be a little hard to get used to if it is not prepared properly to enhance its flavor.

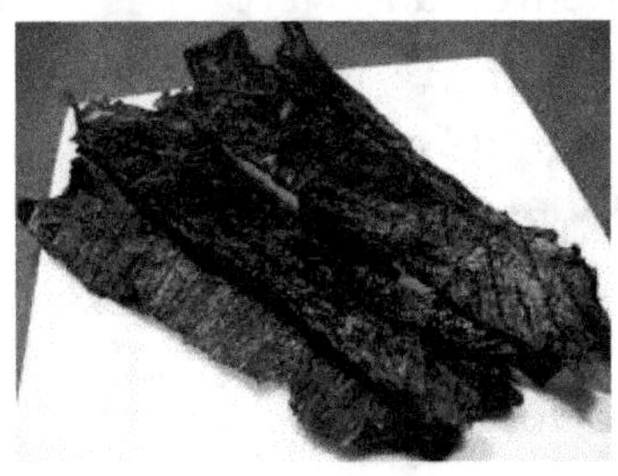

DRIED JERKY

So, you should grind up your excess Venison meat and then go to your butcher and tell him you need some ground beef (or beef fat) to mix with Venison. The butcher will then grind you some beef that has a good fat content.

You should mix the two ground meats together using a 4-to-1 ratio. That is four parts ground Venison and one part fatty ground beef.

I like to add a few other things for more flavor, it's up to you, but I often use; finely ground Onion, maybe a teaspoon or two of my favorite Hot Sauce and even a little Sage, or Minced Rosemary.

Donald W Bobbitt

You can buy artificial or natural casings and once your meat and other ingredients are mixed together well, stuff them into the sausage casings, tie them off and freeze them. Or you can prepare them on the grill, cooking them slowly and thoroughly.

To make sure they are done, I will often partially cook them on one side, and split them open with a knife and then its back onto the grill to finish the cooking.

Other fresh sausages can be made that suit your personal tastes, For example grind up chicken meat and mix with a little sage and onion before stuffing into casings and freezing or cooking.

VINEGAR, Make Your Own

Vinegars can be such a wonderful addition to so many different food dishes that a good chef will usually keep a variety of flavored Vinegars in their pantry, ready to use.

The surprising thing for many people is the fact that making your own flavored Vinegars is such a simple process requiring minimal investment and just a small amount of time.

You can make your vinegars using almost anything that contains Sugar or even Starch. Some of the more popular starter fruits that are often used for vinegars are; almost any Herb, fruit, fruit peelings, and/or fruit juices from such plants as; Apples, Apricots, Blueberries, Carrots, Coconuts, Cranberries, Grapes, Oranges, Pineapple, Persimmons and Peaches to name just a few.

In fact, making a vinegar from more than one fruit and Herb combination can produce some interesting flavors.

NOTE: Be sure that any juices you use are natural and have not been pasteurized or contain any chemicals that can interfere with the fermentation process.

VINEGAR RECIPE:
1. Use a large glass or enamelware pot to start your homemade vinegar.
2. Sterilize the container with boiling water.
3. Wash the fruit and peelings well and add them to the clean pot.
4. Cover the materials in the pot with distilled water.
5. Cover the pot securely with a cheesecloth or other material that is porous and "can breathe". This will allow natural bacteria and yeasts to pass through and start the fermentation process. You can aid this process with an organic starter or even 1/2 cup of "mother" vinegar.

110

6. Set aside and open to stir mixture daily until the odor reaches the intensity of smell and flavor that you want in your homemade vinegar.
7. Strain the liquid from the solids removing as much of the solids as possible.
8. At this point, you can bottle your Vinegar, typically in temporary bottles for the last part of the process.
9. If you want to make a more gourmet style of vinegar you can add other **Herbal flavors**, such as: Basil, Cilantro, Dill, Garlic, Ginger root, Hot Peppers, Lavender, Onions, Oregano, and Thyme.
10. Just fill the temporary bottles with your vinegar and then add the Herb of your choice to the vinegar.
11. Then seal the combination in a bottle, seal it and store it in a cool place to continue working for another 6-weeks.
12. Pour the finished liquid through a filter cloth into a final clean sealable bottle. Any fruit or herbal residue can cause the vinegar to eventually spoil.
13. Label the bottle.

These homemade vinegars can make great seasonal gifts for your friends.

WOOD FLOOR Cleaner

Are your wood floors dull looking? Are they sticky feeling when you walk across them? Are there dark areas of stain buildup in high traffic areas?

If any of these are true you might want to try this recipe for a natural wood floor cleaner that will bring back that glossy look of your wood floors.

RECIPE: Mix together 1-cup of Apple Cider Vinegar, 3-tbs. of Rubbing Alcohol 2-cups of water and 3-4 drops of your favorite Essential Oil for it's scent, such as Pine Oil. Mix well before using.

Use a cloth (or mop?) to rub the liquid onto the floor and it will clean the floor. The dirt should break up, the stains should clear and your wood floor should be brighter looking.

BOOK-2 – Your HEALTH at HOME

This Book includes useful **Tips for the Retro-Survivalist** who wants to take control of the health products that they use in their daily lives and who are interested in expanding their knowledge of the many natural remedies that have been used by people around the world for centuries.

Learn about **Essential Oils** and **Herbs** that have established health and medicinal benefits that you can use in your everyday life. Learn how to make some of your own medicines and how to apply them

Also learn about the many useful tools that you can use to make your daily life not only healthier but also cheaper.

The third book, to be published later will be called **BOOK-3, FOODS, HERBS and Foraging**.

This book is an alphabetical listing of plants foods and herbs that can be cultivated or even found growing wild. Each item will include pictures, descriptions of the plant, its food and/or health uses and suggested medical applications.

This book will provide suggested health and medical applications, both those that have been used for centuries in parts of the world and others that have not been proven but are purported to work.

And there will be a fourth book that I plan to call **BOOK-4, Skills for the Survivalist**. This book will exhibit many of the personal skills that a Survivalist will need in their day-to-day lives, such as construction skills, Tool and Equipment construction skills and Living Crafts.

DOCTORS, PHARMACIES and NATURE

Having good Doctors around, when you are seriously ill is a good thing. Having Pharmacies around to give you the medicines that Doctors prescribe for you, when you are seriously ill, is also a good thing.

You will get no argument from me about both of these being necessary for the world's health.

But, these two things, the world of Physicians and the corporate controlled Pharmacies are technology chasers; they are always racing towards a better cure or a better pill. And, sad to say, they often forget that what they do is for their fellow humans and become driven by their thirst for higher and higher profits.

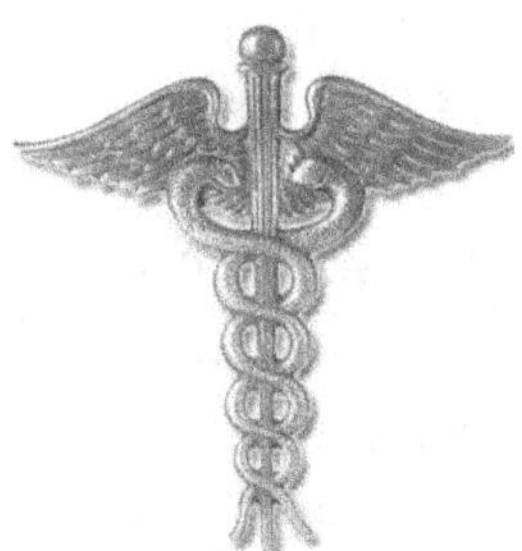

And, they discard those proven "old ways" of treating many of the simple illness' of people and go for the pill with the latest combinations of new chemicals (with their new side effects).

These new pills are so easy to prescribe, dispense, and of course, control their costs and thus increase your profits that natural cures just seem a bother.

But, those natural cures are still here, or at least their ingredients are. The roots that can heal cuts, the flowers that can relieve pain, the tree bark that can lower blood pressure or cholesterol levels, and on and on. They are still here.

We just need to know how to recognize them, find them, and prepare them properly. Oh, I am not saying that we stop going to Doctors, I am saying that your need for most common Doctor visits will decrease, as you learn how to use the still valid natural cures and treatments that our ancestors used.

Apple Cider Vinegar

The old saying "Eat an Apple a Day, and Keep the Doctor Away!" has proven to be more prophetic than anyone ever thought. We have all heard the Apple is a very nutritious fruit that when consumed regularly can provide a great boost to your overall healthy.

Well, it seems that consuming Apple Cider Vinegar has proven to be a healthy habit for people also.

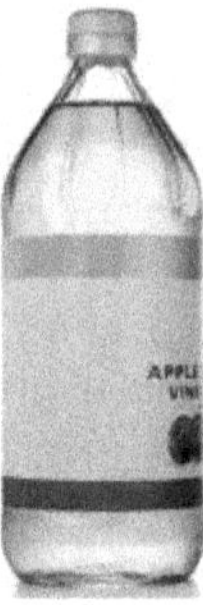

When you use real unpasteurized Apple Cider and ferment it into Apple Cider Vinegar, the sugars are converted into Malic and Acetic Acids. In addition, the Vinegar will contain Pectin's.

The **Malic Acid** gives the Vinegar its distinctive flavor and odor and is key to its bacteria and fungus fighting capabilities. The **Acetic Acid** helps lower the body's blood pH levels thus also helping to fight bacterial infections. The **Pectin** helps lower the body's blood pressure and even lowers Cholesterol levels.

Organic or raw Apple Cider Vinegar is raw, unfiltered, unpasteurized and usually is only about 5% acidic. It will look cloudy and not clear at all. This is considered the best variant of ACV to purchase and use for its health benefits.

You will often see it referenced as **Mother vinegar**.

Mother vinegar contains living bacteria and Enzymes as well as the key nutrients that, when combined, are so good for your health.

Drink ACV Vinegar Safely

If you decide to drink Apple Cider Vinegar, especially the Organic (Mother) variety daily, you should dilute it with water in a ratio of 2-tsp of Vinegar in 8-ounces or more of the other liquid.

If you are worried about your tooth enamel being affected by the

> Avoid drinking ACV with acidic drinks such as; Fruit Juices, Energy drinks, Sodas, etc. It is best to drink it with a meal if possible, to help dilute its high acid level.

acid in the Vinegar, drink the mixture through a straw. Some people also rinse their mouth afterwards with a combination of water and Baking Soda.

Health attributes of Apple Cider Vinegar

Because of its chemical attributes mentioned above, drinking **Apple Cider Vinegar** aids with the following health problems:

- Fights allergies,
- Aids in healing respiratory infections,
- Acts as a disinfectant on the skin and thus helps get rid of Warts and Acne
- Lowers blood sugar levels,
- Lowers Cholesterol and Triglyceride levels,
- Is a mild laxative,
- Relieves sinus congestion,
- Reduce gas and bloating,
- Reduce leg cramps,
- Aids in reducing the chance of Kidney stones
- Includes Amino Acids which boosts the metabolism,
- Includes Malic Acid which helps reduce clogged arteries
- Soothes a sore throat,
- Increases enzyme production, which helps the body digest fats.
- Aids in reducing weight over time.

As can be seen by this extensive list, Apple Cider Vinegar is a powerful natural tool that an individual can use to maintain a healthy body.

HERBAL TEAS – For your Health

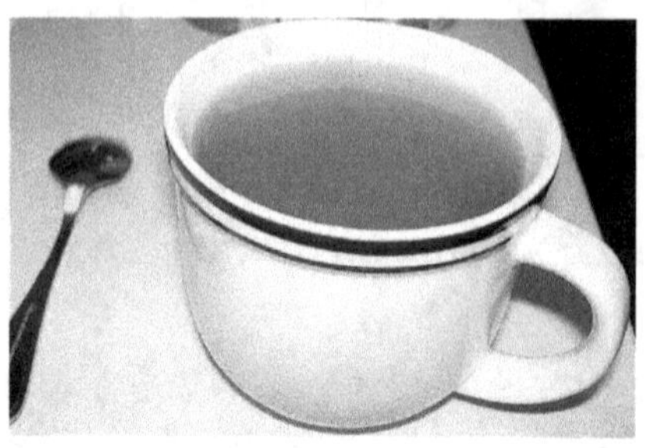

The use of Tea as a healthy beverage has a history that goes back for thousands of years around the world.

Many types of tea plants have been cultivated over time for very specific health qualities and their specific flavors.

The **four major types** of tea plants that are cultivated around the world today are:

BLACK Tea: Black Tea gets its name from the black color of its leaves after they are oxidized. It is also known as Red Tea in the Far East and is made from the leaves of the Assamese plant.

The picked tea leaves are allowed to wither and are then crushed to release the Oils. Then they are dried for specifically four hours before the tea is packaged.

OOLONG Tea: Oolong Tea is the more traditional Chinese variety of teas. The Chinese name actually means Black Dragon Tea in English.

The leaves and buds are dried in the Sun until they are withered and oxidized. It is roasted for anywhere from 12 to 36 hours. At this point, the leaves are rolled in one of two ways; either into long curly leaves or small beads.

GREEN Tea: Green Tea is made by minimizing oxidation of the leaves during the production process and generally Green Teas have the highest levels of Polyphenols.

There is a wide variation in the distribution of Green Tea around the world. Often, this is due to the wide range of manufacturing processes used around the world, and which brands and types are made available.

WHITE TEA: White Tea is made from the young leaves and unopened buds on the tea plant. It is called White Tea due to the light coloring of the strands on the unopened buds. The leaves are withered in the Sun and only lightly oxidized to protect their flavor.

In addition to consuming beverages made from the leaves of the Tea plant itself, over time people have used certain other herbs in their teas to provide specific nutrients and even medical aid for some human ailments.

Herbal Teas (or **Infusions**) are usually relatively strong compared to what is in your standard tea bag.

Tea Making Tips

Whenever possible make your tea with loose tea rather than tea bags. Many people do not realize that the tea in tea bags is of inferior quality to the loose product that can be purchased on the web and in specialty stores.

Basic Tea Recipe

A typical and simple Herbal Tea would be made of 1-ounce or more of your dried herbal tea mixture and 1-quart of hot water.

Using higher quality teas means that you are getting a richer flavor along with increased health benefits from the unsullied raw ingredients. For this reason, tea bags should only be used for their relative convenience when making your day-to-day variety teas.

Do Not overheat your tea

Excessive heat can often destroy the medicinal power and even the flavor of the final product by causing the loss of much of the critical ingredients that you desired the tea for anyway.

The water used for Tea should be brought to a boil and then allowed to sit and drop below the boiling temperature for a few minutes before adding the tea.

You can purchase the appropriate kitchen herbs, medicinal herbs and teas to make your own special herbal teas in specialty stores, herb stores. Health food stores and even on the web.

The number of possible ingredient combinations for making your own herbal tea is almost endless so, below are some of the more popular herbal teas, and which ailments they can be used to treat;

CHAMOMILE Tea with Lavender

Chamomile Tea has a history that goes back for hundreds of years as a flavorful tea to sip on, enjoy its flavors and relax with in the evening or before bedtime.

Chamomile has an Apple-like flavor and its name is the Greek word for "ground Apples". There are two plant varieties, the German and the Roman, but the flowers of the German variety is the more potent and thus is the preferred for tea.

This tea will help **settle the stomach**, is a **relaxant** and can help **induce sleep**. The added Lavender provides a pleasing, relaxing aroma. This Tea is also said to ease **muscle pains** and **menstrual cramps**.

RECIPE: For each cup of tea you should;
1. Mix 2-tbs of dried Chamomile flowers with 1-tsp of dried Lavender buds. Crush them together well and then place the mixture into a tea bag or strainer and add 2-cups of hot water.
2. Allow the mixture to steep for typically 2-3 minutes, or longer if you want your tea stronger.
3. Or, you can pour the hot water over your loose tea leaves in a pot and allow the mixture to steep and then pour it through a sieve or strainer placed over the teacup.
4. Sweeten the tea with Honey, if desired. The Lavender is said to cure headaches and relieve anxiety.

Chamomile Tea Health Benefits

Here is a list of the medicinal benefits attributed to Chamomile and thus to Chamomile Tea;

It is a **mild sedative** and **anti-bacterial** that fights; **arthritic pain, colds, indigestion, infections, joint inflammation, stomach cramps, menstrual cramps and reduces tension.**

ELDERBERRY FLOWER Tea

Elderberries themselves are considered a great Influenza treatment and you can also make a nice tea from the flowers that can provide interesting health benefits.

Drinking a couple of cups of Elderberry Tea can **help fight off both Type A and B forms of Influenza.** Elderberries and the flowers are high in **antioxidants** and are a good **anti-inflammatory.**

RECIPE: You can make Elderberry Tea by soaking the flowers in warm water for up to 10 hours. Then, sift the flowers from the liquid before warming it properly and drinking the tea itself.

GINGER TEA

Ginger Tea is good for treating common **colds** and it can be made by using the following recipe:

- Chop Ginger Root into small squares and pound the squares until they are a "mush".
- Add ½ cup of this to four cups of water and bring the mixture to a low boil.
- Boil the mixture for about five minutes and then strain the liquid into a jar. (This liquid can be kept for several days in a fridge.).
- When ready to use it, bring the mixture to a near boil, pour it into a cup and allow it to sit and cool for a few minutes before drinking it.

When drinking Ginger tea you can add a little honey or Lemon to improve the taste.

HAWTHORN BERRY Tea

Hawthorn Berries are actually a healthy food in their own right, but they can also be used to make a Tea that is not only nutritious but also healthy.

Hawthorn Berries are high in **antioxidants** and other key nutrients. Made into a tea or tonic, they are safely used to treat; **angina, arteriosclerosis, cardiac arrhythmia, congestive heart failure**, and **high blood pressure** and **myocarditis**.

Hawthorn Tea RECIPE:
- Crush and add ½-cup of hawthorn berries (in a bag) to a quart of water in a saucepan.
- Bring the water to a boil and then reduce the heat and allow the mixture to simmer for 20-minutes.
- Remove from the heat and allow it to steep for 10-minutes and then drink.

HIBISCUS Tea

Hibiscus (*sabdariffa*) flowers are high in **antioxidants** and contain **anthocyanin** and are often used to make the popular Hibiscus fruit drinks consumed in some countries as well as by many people to make an herbal tea.

Hibiscus Tea has a citrus-like flavor and aids in **lowering blood pressure in Diabetics**, and others with **mild hypertension**.

Hibiscus Tea RECIPE:

- Add ½-cup of dried and crushed Hibiscus flowers (in a bag) to 1-quart of hot water.
- Allow it to steep for about 10-minutes before drinking.

LAVENDER Tea

Lavender Tea has its own powerful aroma and a unique flavor, but people will often drink it for its ability to; **relieve the pain of headaches** and **reduces stress**.

Lavender is a very popular addition to many herbal teas because of the wonderful aroma it imparts to the tea.

Lavender Tea RECIPE:

- To make 1-cup of Lavender Tea.
- Add 2-tbs of finely chopped fresh Lavender flowers (in a bag) to 1-cup of boiling water.
- Allow it to step for 10-minutes.
- Remove the bag.
- Add Honey to sweeten before drinking.

LEMON BALM Tea

Fresh Lemon Balm leaves have a lemony flavor and aroma and are used to make lemon balm tea.

> CAUTION: Be aware that **using lemon balm can interfere with hypothyroid medications** and is sometimes used as an herbal treatment for hyperthyroidism.

Lemon Balm Tea is often consumed because of its ability to **ease headaches** as well as for **easing anxiety and depression**.

Lemon Balm Tea RECIPE: To make a cup of Lemon Balm Tea;
- Chop up enough of the fresh leaves of the Lemon Balm plant to make 2-tbs of a mush.
- Place this into a bag and add to 1-cup of boiling water.
- Allow the mixture to steep for 5-minutes.
- Then remove the bag and drink the tea.

LINDEN FLOWER Tea

Linden Tea is made from the sweet smelling flowers of the Linden tree. The flowers can be bought and used as desired or you can purchase and grow your own tree. Then you can collect and dry the flowers yourself.

The Tea is very nutritious and provides a number of health benefits including; reducing **anxiety**, reducing the pain of **headaches**, easing **insomnia** due to its **sedative** properties, helps the body fight bacteria, helps fight **asthma**, and **bronchitis**.

Linden Tea can also **aid the digestive system** by fighting **diarrhea** and **stomach cramps**.

Linden Tea RECIPE:
- Add 2-3 tbs. of chopped, dried Linden flowers (in a bag) to about a quart of boiling water.
- Remove the heat and allow the mixture to steep for five minutes.
- Remove the bag of flowers and
- Enjoy the Tea. Add a little Honey to sweeten the tea.

RED CLOVER Tea

Red Clover can be cultivated, but it grows wild in many parts of the world. The bright red blooms have a sweet honey-like odor but the tea has very little flavor. The dried flowers can be used to make a very nutritious and healthy Tea.

Red Clover is a rich source of **isoflavones**, which act like **estrogen**. Red Clover Tea is used to treat such problems as: **PMS, Hot Flashes** and **High Cholesterol**.

It is also used to improve **urine production** and **blood production**, as well as to reduce the possibility of **osteoporosis**. It can act like a **blood thinner** and reduce the possibility of **blood clots and arterial plaques**. The Tea is also good for treating **Colds** and a **Sore Throat**.

Red Clover Tea RECIPE:
- Add 2-3 cups of whole, dried Red Clover flowers (in a bag) to one quart of boiling water.
- Remove the heat and cover.
- Then allow the mixture to steep for five minutes,
- Remove the bag of flowers and enjoy the Tea.
- Add a little Honey to take the edge off and sweeten the tea.

There is a Red Clover Tea concoction that includes adding Dandelion or Plantain Leaf. This tea is nourishing and has a relatively high Calcium and Iron content.

Some women use it to promote a **healthy Lymphatic system** and **Reproductive system,** *particularly the* **breasts**. Drinking this tea

Due to the weak flavor of Red Clover Tea you might want to add a little of one of your other favorite and more flavorful teas, such as Chamomile, to the mixture when preparing the tea.

is purported to also help with **menstrual cramps.**

Respiratory aid - Regularly drinking Red Clover tea, with the addition of a drop of **Yellow Dock** and a Peppermint leaf is said to help in reducing the severity of cases of **Asthma, Colds** and other **respiratory problems.**

ROSEMARY Tea with LAVENDER

Rosemary the flavorful herb used by so many chefs in so many dishes also makes a great tea that is often used to provide relief from Headaches.

RECIPE: How to make one cup of Rosemary Tea.

Chop up the leaves and even the blooms of the Rosemary plant to make one tbs. of a mash. Place this into a bag and place the bag in boiling water, remove it from the heat and allow it to steep for about 10-minutes.

Pour and drink the tea to relieve a **headache**. Add Lemon Balm and Honey to lighten the strong Rosemary flavor.

SPICE TEA or MASALA CHAI

Spice Tea, also known as Masala Chai Tea is actually made with a variety of spices around the world.

The predominant spices used are; Bay Leaves, Cardamom, Cinnamon, Cloves, Coriander, Fennel Seed, Ginger, Lemon Grass and Peppermint, to name just a few.

The inclusion of this mixture of spices in your daily tea will **provide a therapeutic boost to your body in its fight against common colds.**

Other Herbal Teas

There are literally hundreds of Herbal Tea blends consumed around the world and many of them not only taste wonderful but many also have valuable healing properties.

The serious herbal tea aficionado should research these other lesser-known plants and herbs and the teas that can be made from them.

Here are just a few of these Tea varieties and their healthful benefits;
- **Cinnamon – High Cholesterol, anti-viral, anti-bacterial,**
- **Meadowsweet - pain relief, stomach problems .**

- **Peppermint** – Sore Throat, colds, heartburn, nausea.
- **Rooibos** - antioxidant, anti-inflammatory, Diabetes, Insomnia.
- And many more.

Flavoring an HERBAL TEA

Often, an herbal tea may taste strong or even be unsavory. When this is the case, you can add certain spices and other ingredients to subdue the original flavors of the tea without harming its health benefits.

Cinnamon flavoring – Cinnamon can be used to make a nutritious and healthy tea by itself, but its unique flavor makes it a great addition for many other herbal teas.

Honey flavoring – Honey is the sweetener of choice for most teas. Honey not only sweetens but also has its own healthy properties.

Mint flavoring – Many people enjoy the refreshing flavor that a leaf of Peppermint, or other natural mint, can add to their favorite herbal tea.

Lemon Peel flavoring or Orange Peel flavoring – Add a Lemon or Orange Peel twist to your Herbal Tea to impart a great citrusy fruit flavor.

FORAGING – What to look for

There are so many plants growing wild in your back yard, in parks, in forests and even along roadsides that can, not only provide sustenance but many of them have been used for centuries as health aids and some are even to cure illnesses.

And, over the centuries, people would forage for most of these plants when they needed them.

For one thing, these plants were not just used for eating but many were used as spices or for treating certain medical problems.

Because only a small amount of these plants was needed to treat a health problem, only a small amount was collected at a time allowing the remaining plants to be there for use another day.

The key to foraging is that **you must know what you are looking for** as well as know when to look. Foraging is a lost art for many of us because it has not been passed down to the new generations of people, as was once done in families.

In todays society such rural skills have been long lost and replaced by the conveniences of living in cities.

> **CAUTION:** Foraging for safe and useful wild plants is something that must be taught, in the field, and not just learned from a book.

Take the time to study these plants and get into foraging yourself for some very valuable medicinal goods that are out there just waiting to be found.

If you are serious about foraging, then you should first **learn what grows wild** in the area where you live. Check around with your friends and seek out anyone who has knowledge or experience in Foraging. There is probably an experienced forager living near you so contact them and have them teach you what is out there growing wild locally, just waiting for you.

A beginner Forager should take their cameras with them and collect pictures of plants and then, when you are home, you can use these to research whether these plants are safe to eat or use medicinally.

Becoming a successful Forager is going to take a lot of time, just walking around and discovering and learning about what nature has waiting for you.

You need to learn what a potentially valuable plant looks like, but you will also need to learn about things like; where they flourish, when they should be collected and what companion plants grow in the same types of sites.

You must also learn to **trust your sense of smell**. Often the odor of a plant can be critical when trying to determine if you have the plant you want, or maybe just a look-alike.

The smart forager also needs to know the plant's structure and recognize which parts are actually safe to use.

Although some plants have edible parts or parts useful for health or with medicinal applications, always be aware that there are some plants which **have toxic parts** as well as parts that are useful.

Harvesting:

If you do find a unique or rare plant growing in an area, do not over harvest the area. Leave most of the plants to grow and propagate for future years of collection and use.

It is recommended that you only harvest 5-10% of an area's plant growth to assure that it will continue to thrive for future harvesting.

Of course, once you find one of these treasures of nature, you should go back and learn how the plant itself looks during all of the seasons. This will help you find the particular plant more easily throughout the year.

One other note, the plant you want to forage, regardless of what it might be, must look, feel and taste healthy when you do collect samples if it, Always be aware that **a plant can catch diseases** and have **fungus growths**, just as humans do, and these should not be used if they do not look healthy.

Toxic Plants

Toxic plants grow everywhere in the USA and are always to be avoided.

You should understand that if you are foraging near population centers, there is always a chance that the pretty flower you see growing wild was once domesticated.

But regardless of whether they are domesticated or not, some of these plants have edible parts and some are going to be toxic.

One should NEVER, NEVER eat a part of a plant unless they are ABSOLUTELY 100% POSITIVE that they know what they are eating.

There are too many plants out there that look just alike and one can be edible while the other can be deadly, such as the **Wild Carrot** and the **Hemlock** plants as examples.

In **Table-B2-1 Foraging for Plants – the Good and the Bad**, you will see a partial list of many plants that have edible parts and some that have parts of the plant that are not edible.

The list is nowhere near complete, but it is a pretty good start for someone who is interested in Foraging.

Old Sayings about Foraging

There are several great old folk saying about eating certain plants found in the wild and here are a few;

Leaves of three? Let it be! – This is actually true of Poison Ivy and Poison Oak along with several other 3-leaf plants you may come upon in your travels through the wild, but there are also some 3-leaf plants that are OK to eat.

No to Milky Sap! – Old folk stories will tell you to avoid eating plants that have a milky sap, and this is actually true of the majority of these plants with their milky colored sap, but again, there are some exceptions that are safe to consume.

If animals can eat it, so can you? – This one is generally true but some plants that animals will eat are not OK for humans to eat. For instance, animals eat acorns, but acorns should be soaked in water for several hours to remove the high concentration of **Tannin** in them, before humans can safely eat them without getting sick.

The point here is that there are far too many differences in plant varieties for people to make generalized statements about the safety of one plant characteristic over another about a plants safety for human consumption.

There are even cases of, when some plants, in different stages of it's growth can have far different affects on the person consuming or using them

For instance; some plants are only edible after they have wilted, some plants are only edible after they have been dried, some plants and seeds are only poisonous after they have mixed with the digestive juices in the stomach, and some are only edible when they are young.

This list goes on, but the point is, ALWAYS BE SURE before you eat a new plant that you are not sure of.

TOXIC Symptoms

Again, there is only one standard you must follow when foraging to assure that you will not be poisoned; If you are NOT 100% SURE that a plant is safe then DO NOT EAT IT!

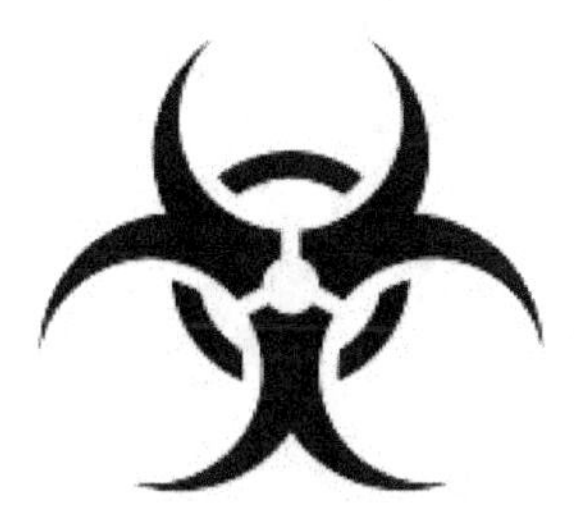

And, if you suspect that you or someone else has eaten a plant that might be poisonous you should always note the symptoms, collect a sample of the plant and consult a physician.

Toxic plant symptoms typically are one or more of these listed below:

Vomiting, Stomach pains, Skin irritation, and **an irregular heartbeat, burning in the mouth**, even **possibly Convulsions or Seizures.**

The severity of the symptoms can vary widely depending on the plant and the quantity consumed and the size of the person who ate the plant.

NOTE: For a **skin irritation**, quickly wash the areas affected with water and for the eyes thoroughly irrigate them with clean water for 15-20 minutes.

NOTE: If the plant was **swallowed, rinse out the person's mouth** immediately and take them to a nearby hospital or Poison Centre. And, of course, **take a sample of the plant** with you.

NOTE: Always, always contact a physician immediately if there is any doubt about the potential danger from what you have eaten or touched.

Seasonal Plant Harvesting

Generally speaking, the important parts of an edible plants structure will be ready for harvesting during certain seasons of the year.

These plant parts and the pertinent seasons are shown in the table below:

General Plant Harvesting Seasons				
	Spring	Summer	Fall	Winter
Leave s	xxx	xxx		
Roots			Late	xxx
Fruits		Late	xxx	
Seeds		Late	xxx	

Mushrooms – The GOOD and the BAD

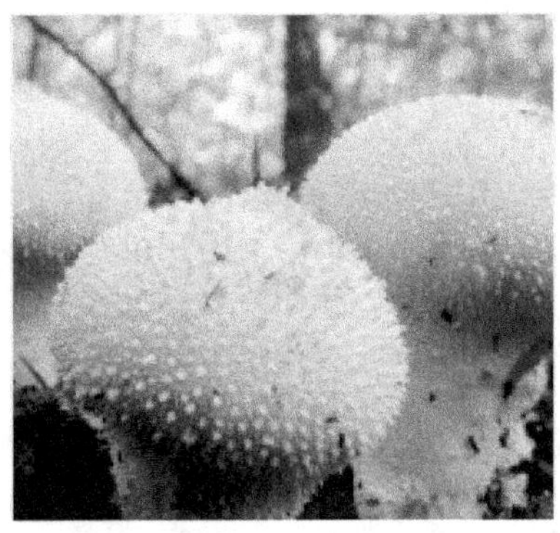

Edible wild

BOVIST Mushroom

Mushrooms (AKA toadstools) are actually classified as fungi and many of them are prized for their fantastic flavors when used in cooking and there are even a small number that are prized for their health properties.

Mushrooms are relatively easily cultivated and many of the edible varieties are available in supermarkets and can be found, in season, at farmers markets.

Edible Mushrooms are a great source of B Vitamins, Antioxidants and such minerals as Selenium, Potassium and Copper.

But, even though there are **over 10,000 species** of Mushrooms growing wild in the US, there are **only around 250 of them that are safe and edible.**

Mushroom Toxins:

Many mushrooms contain toxins that can have very debilitating effects on the human body, and there are some that can even cause death within 2 to 6 days after ingestion if the person is not treated properly.

Types of mushroom toxins.

The first type is **Protoplasmic Toxins** and these can destroy certain human cells and even lead to organ failure.

The second types are called **Neurotoxins**. These can cause such reactions as: convulsions, hallucinations, depression, excessive sweating and even a coma.

The third types are **Gastro-intestinal Irritants**. These can produce such symptoms as: nausea, diarrhea, vomiting and even abdominal cramps.

The fourth type, are what are called ***Disulfiram*-like toxins** which have specific toxic symptoms if alcohol is consumed within 72-hours after eating these mushrooms. The symptoms will occur within 15-minutes of consuming alcohol. The list of **symptoms** when poisoning does occur includes; **flushing of the skin, unusual drowsiness, metallic taste in mouth, severe stomach pain** and a **drop in blood pressure**.

Popular Commercial Mushrooms

Of course, if you are worried about your mushroom collecting skills, you can always go to your supermarket and grab a package of one of the many popular cultivated varieties of mushrooms available, such as; **Button-top, Shitake Mushrooms** and **Portobello** to name a few. And, of course, you can safely consume these commercially cultivated mushrooms.

Foraging for Mushrooms:

But, when it comes to foraging in the wild for Mushrooms, you need to be very careful or you could easily end up poisoning yourself and even your family and friends.

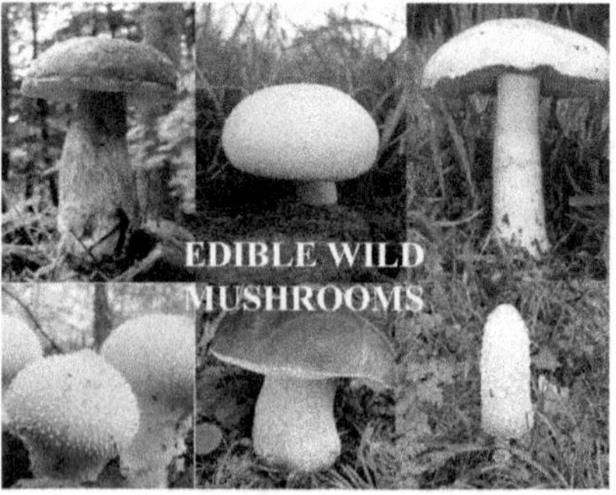

 In fact, it is not recommended to forage for mushrooms in the wild at all if you are not a trained expert at this unique skill.

The identification of a "safe" mushroom entails the consideration of such things as; odors, shades of color, habitat, season and even bruising reactions in order to define one variety of mushroom from another.

So if you are not properly trained you should stay away from any unknown variety you may come upon in the wild.

There are several mushrooms that are popular for foraging that are safe for the experienced Mushroom hunter to eat and some of these are; the **Bay Bolete**, the **Bovist mushroom**, the **Field Mushroom**, the **Horse Mushroom**, the **Penny Bun** and the **Shaggy Ink Cap**, to name just a few.

Mushroom Collecting Tips

If you do want to learn how to safely collect mushrooms yourself, it is recommended that you check around locally and see if you can find someone who is experienced at collecting mushrooms.

If you can, go out with them and have them show you which ones you can collect safely and more importantly how they find the safe ones as well as what criteria they used to find, examine and confirm the safety of these specific mushrooms.

Handling Mushrooms

Just a few other hints for the collector,

1- Keep ALL of your collected mushrooms separated until you are home and have confirmed whether each variety collected is safe or not.
2- Do not bruise your mushrooms as they will go bad much faster if they are bruised,
3- Refrigerate your collected mushrooms when you do get home because they will keep fresh longer if kept cold.

And, once again: DO NOT CONSUME ANY MUSHROOM that you are not 100% confident it is a safe, edible mushroom.

Mushrooms for Medical Applications

Now, I will list several mushrooms that are purported to provide some specific health benefits for some people. Some of them are even used to treat certain cancer conditions in parts of the world.

Some mushrooms have been used, literally for thousands of years, to treat certain serious illnesses, mostly due to the fact that they have very **strong immune system boosting properties** as well as high levels of antioxidants that help the body fight some malignant cancerous tumors.

CHAGA Mushrooms

The Chaga Mushroom is a large and ugly black growth found

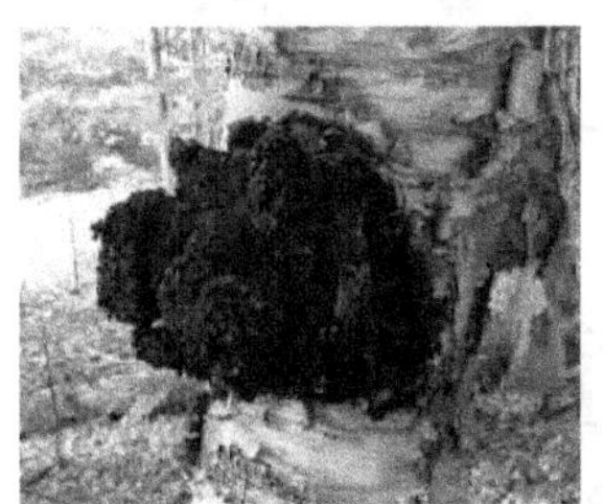

mostly on Yellow and White Birch trees in the colder northern regions of Europe, Russia, Asia and North America.

This mushroom is very dense with a cracked surface and is usually brittle and tends to flake away when you try to remove it.

Once removed from the tree, it is best to break it up into small pieces and then dry these and make them into a powder for storage and later use.

Dry them at 110-115F for 24-hours and then set them aside for several days and repeat the drying process again to make sure the interior moisture is totally removed.

Then run the pieces through a grinder to make a powder.

It has been used as a folk medicine for centuries in Russia, specifically in Teas, as a coffee substitute and for its medicinal properties.

Although still under study in the US, an extract of Chaga (known as fraction 1O4) has been **used to actually kill certain cancer cells**

LION's MANE Mushroom

This mushroom is large and white with long hair-like fronds. It grows on trees in Eastern Europe and when cooked it has a flavor similar to Lobster.

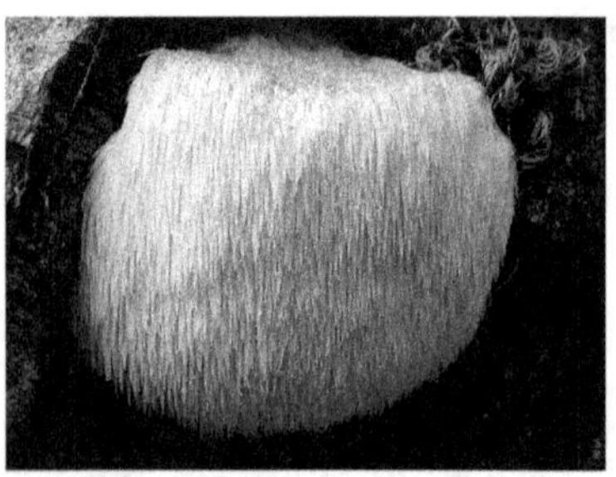

Lion's Mane has been used in folk medicine for hundreds of years. It has been shown to **enhance the body's immune system** and has been used to **assist in the fight against the damaging effects of certain chemotherapy medicines.**

Its use is purported to **aid in treating Multiple Sclerosis and Dementia**. This mushroom helps by increasing the level of Myelin in the brain and aids in clearing up the amyloid plaques associated with Alzheimer's.

It is still undergoing studies but an extract has been shown to help some **cancer patients live longer** and an extract given to lab rats with **colon cancer** have shown regression of the cancers.

OYSTER MUSHROOMS

The Oyster Mushroom (aka; Abalone, Tree Mushroom, Pleurotis) is one of the most popular cultivated mushrooms in the world and is a popular culinary ingredient in dishes such as stir-fry and sauté.

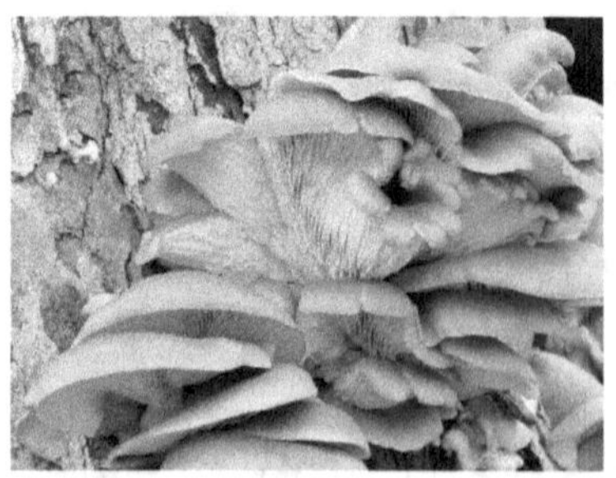

Typically the chef will tear the mushroom apart before cooking rather than cutting them. It is a tree-rot fungi that grows on the trunks of hardwood trees in tropical and temperate zones.

Oyster Mushrooms contain Lovastatin, which is a proven treatment for lowering the body's Cholesterol levels.

The problem is that the levels of dried Oyster Mushrooms that must be consumed by animals to lower Cholesterol levels significantly would be in the range of 5% to 10% of the daily diet.

Regardless, even eating them in the much lower quantities of a cooked dish would be of some help in lowering Cholesterol to some degree.

PORTOBELLO Mushrooms

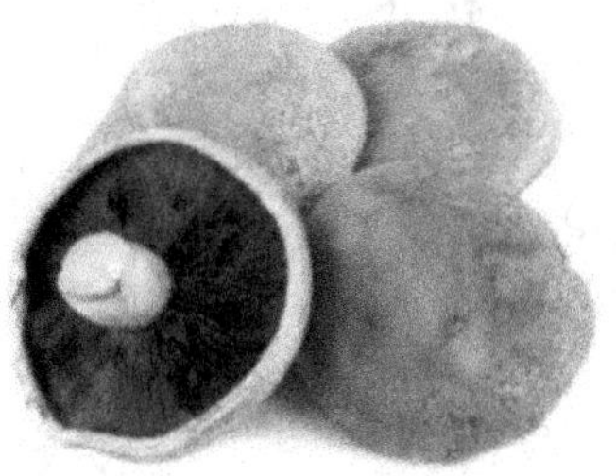

The Portobello is a very popular mushroom; often cultivated and used around the world in food dishes.

The Portobello has a wonderful flavor and a meat-like texture that makes it a favorite ingredient in numerous recipes around the world.

NOTE: Some medical studies have shown that an isolate from the Portobello was proven to be effectively **toxic to some human cancer cells** under laboratory conditions.

REISHI Mushrooms

The Reishi Mushroom, also known as *ganoderma lucidum*, is popular in Japan and China and can generally be found in warmer climates growing on dead and rotting wood.

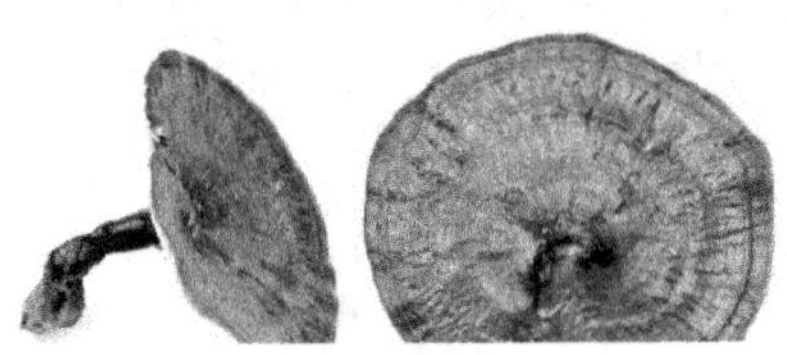

REISHI Mushrooms

The mushroom has **anti-inflammatory**, **anti-viral** and **antioxidant** properties.

Extracts from the Reishi mushroom are reputed to help **protect the Liver** and help **protect the Kidneys** during treatments.

It is purported to aid in **Liver detoxification**, and **lowering blood pressure** and **lowering cholesterol levels.**

It is also effective in **improving the body's immune system** and in **fighting certain forms of cancer** and **fighting HIV**

For some people it also works well in **reducing chemotherapy nausea** and can help increase some other **cancer treatment drugs'** effectiveness, as well as radiation therapy.

SHITAKE Mushrooms

The ever popular Shitake Mushrooms are more than just a delicious ingredient used in many food recipes.

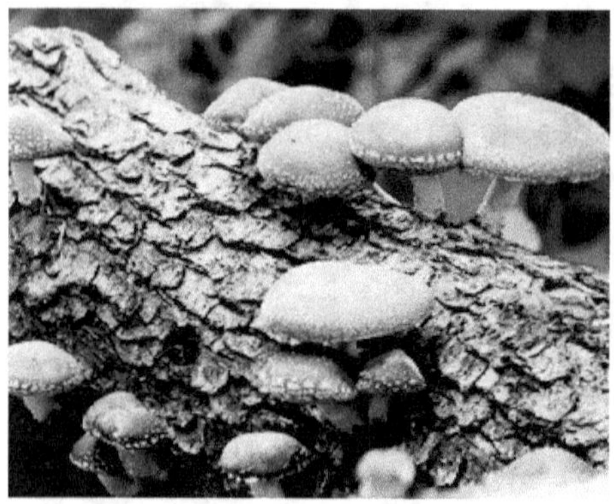

They also have certain health attributes that are being investigated further in a number of scientific medical studies.

Shitake mushrooms contain two chemicals that are of interest to scientists. These are; AHCC and Eritadenine.

AHCC is an extracted compound that has been shown to boost the body's immune system and helps fight Cancer and destroys certain Viruses.

Eritadenine, on the other hand, has been shown to lower Cholesterol in animals and is expected to do the same for humans.

TURKEY TAIL Mushrooms

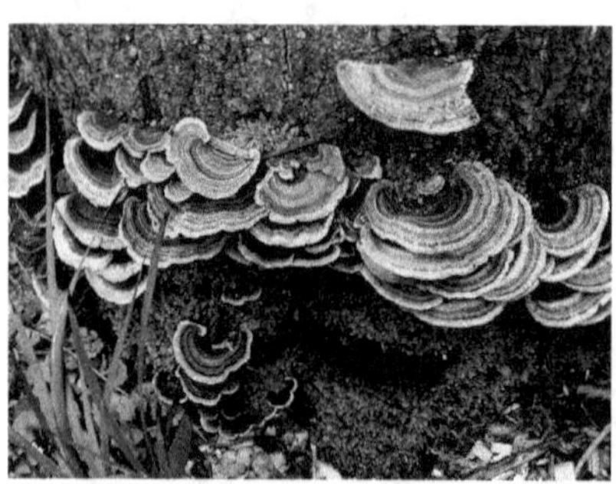

TURKEY TAIL Mushrooms

The Turkey Tail Mushroom is an abundant one that typically grows wild on dead stumps around the world.

It is multi-colored and fan-shaped which is where this mushroom gets its name, as it resembles a spread turkey's tail. Its scientific name is *trametes versicolor*.

These mushrooms grow abundantly and are available at reasonable prices from many sources.

Some companies have studied this mushroom and developed isolates (one is called *Polysaccharide-K*) from it and certain other mushrooms can be **stimulant** for the bodies immune system and prolong the lives of some cancer patients.

It should be noted that there have been cures of some cancer tumors including breast cancer tumors by using the products made from the complete mushroom, which are produced by **Fungi Perfecti**, a noted organic mushroom medicine production company.

Are there other mushrooms out there that can help us lead a healthier life? There are a lot of scientists wondering the same thing and there are a number of them under investigation.

Other Healthy Fungi

There are forms of Fungi that produce chemicals that have proven as significant for treating certain Health conditions.

Cyclosporine:

A fungi known as *Cordyceps subsessilis* is a parasite of Beetles and contains **Cyclosporine** which is an effective **immune-suppressant** and is used to treat such conditions as; transplant rejection, psoriasis, rheumatoid arthritis, Crohn's Disease and ulcerative colitis, among others.

Make your own Healthy POULTICE

A Poultice is a handy medicinal tool that can be used for treating health problems that are painful, aching, inflamed or infected.

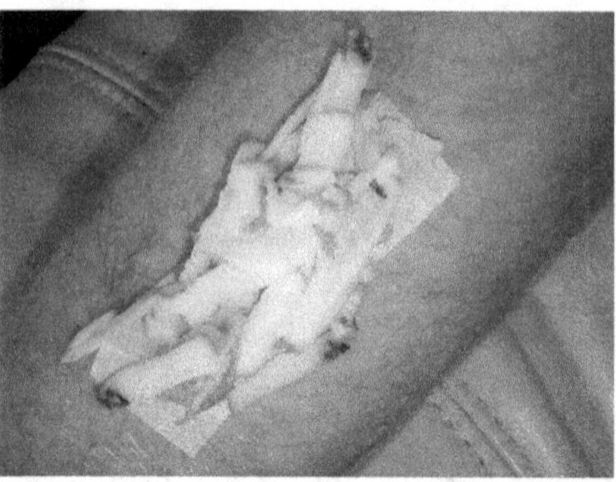

A poultice typically consists of a moist mass of crushed and chopped herbs, plants, and oils, normally mixed with warm water.

Then they are usually wrapped in a sterile yet porous cloth that is placed over the wounded or affected area of the skin.

Some of the health problems that can be treated with poultices are; **Abscesses, Boils, Chest Congestion, Hemorrhoids, Earaches, Infections**, and **Inflammations**. Here are a few popular and effective poultices:

Cayenne Pepper Poultice

Cayenne Pepper is a **great Styptic**, so it can be applied directly to a cut to **stop bleeding.** It is also a great **anti-bacterial** and **pain reliever** when used in a Poultice.

Used to Treat: **bleeding, Arthritic Pain, Sore Muscles, Sprains** and more.

RECIPE: First, mix ½-tsp. of Cayenne Pepper powder with a little vegetable oil, or water, to make a paste. Wrap the paste in a thin cloth and apply directly over the affected area. Wrap or tape the poultice to hold it in place and change the poultice 2-3 times a day.

Comfrey Poultice

Comfrey is a great herb that is used to **aid in the healing of Broken Bones and Sprains and even for simple Cuts and Bruises.**

RECIPE: To make a small poultice simply chop up fresh Comfrey leaves until you have about 2-tbs of the mash. Add a couple of drops of vegetable oil (Olive oil?) to this and 1-tsp of a thickening agent such as flour or ground bran.

Blend the mixture together well and wrap it in a thin sterile cloth and apply the poultice to the wounded area. Wrap or tape the poultice firmly in place. Change the poultice every day until the area is healed.

Jewel Weed Poultice

Jewel Weed is a plant that's widely used to **treat such skin problems as Poison Ivy rashes**.

RECIPE: To make a poultice chop and mash the fresh Jewel Weed leaves together for 2-tbs. of mash. Add these to 1-tsp. of Wood Ash and 2- drops of Linseed Oil. Blend everything together well until it is the consistency of a paste.

Wrap the paste in a thin cloth then wipe a thin layer of Aloe Vera onto the affected area of the skin and apply the poultice directly over this. Wrap or tape the poultice to keep it in place.

Replace the poultice daily.

Lemon Balm Poultice

Lemon Balm is a good **anti-bacterial** and a Lemon Balm poultice is good for treating; **Cold Sores, Insect Bites** and other **Small wounds**.

RECIPE: Mix 1-tsp. of Lemon Balm with a couple of tsp. of warm water to make a thin paste. Wrap the paste in a thin sterile cloth and apply it to the affected area for a couple of hours.

Mustard Poultice

Mustard Seeds are not only nutritious, they are a strong **anti-fungal**, they are **a good source of Omega-3s**. They are also used o treat a number of illnesses and physical problems, such as; **Asthma, blood pressure,** reducing the symptoms of **rheumatoid arthritis,** reducing **migraine headaches,** and in **treating cancers**

RECIPE: Mix 2-tbs. of Mustard Seeds into 1-cup of warm water. Allow the mixture to set for 15-minutes and then remove the now soaked Mustard seeds. Wrap the seeds in a soft cloth and apply this poultice to the affected area.

CAUTION: This **poultice can burn**, so be sure to place a thin cloth between the poultice and the skin.

Onion Poultice

Onion is an **anti-inflammatory** and an **anti-viral** so it is often used to treat such problems as: **Boils** and **Chest Congestion.**

RECIPE: First, chop and mash one small raw onion and mix it with 1-cup of warm water and allow the mixture to sit for 30-minutes.

Pour the mixture through a sieve and wrap the onion mash onto a sterile porous cloth and apply the poultice to the affected area. Change the poultice a couple of times a day for 2-3 days.

Plantain Poultice

The Plantain is a fruit high in **antioxidants** as well as **carotenes**. It can be used to treat; **anemia, neuritis, fights infections and helps reduce constipation.**

RECIPE: Chop up 2-tbs. of fresh Plantain weed, add 1-2-tsp. of vegetable oil to moisten the mixture and wrap in a thin cloth to apply to the affected area. Add ½-tsp. of activated charcoal to increase its drawing power. This poultice is a good treatment for Insect bites and stings.

Potato Poultice

RECIPE: Chop and grind up 1-cup of raw potato and soak it in sterile warm water for 10-minutes. Remove the potato mash and wrap it in a sterile soft cloth.

Place the poultice over the affected area and wrap or tape it to the body to hold it in place.

This poultice is good to use as an **anti-inflammatory** and works well for **treating Eye infections and other infections.** Of course, you want to place the poultice over the closed eye.

Slippery Elm and Thyme Poultice

Because Slippery Elm has **strong healing properties** and Thyme is a **very good antiseptic**; they work together well in a poultice to treat such problems as **Boils** and **infections in cuts.**

RECIPE: Chop and crush 2-3 Thyme leaves and add it to 1-cup of boiling water and then allow to sit for 10-minutes. Remove the leaves and add to 2-tbs.of Slippery Elm powder. Add a few drops of vegetable oil (Olive Oil?), if necessary to make a nice paste.

Wrap the paste in a thin cloth and apply to the affected area for up to 2-hours.

Tea Tree Oil Poultice

Tea Tree Oil is good for treating: **Skin Infections, Rashes** and **Poison Ivy, Poison Oak** and **Poison Sumac.**

Recipe for Tee Tree Oil Poultice:

Place 1-tsp. Of Tea Tree Oil in ¼- cup of hot water and allow it to sit for 10-minutes, Add 2-tbs. of Baking Soda and ¼-tsp. of Salt.

Blend the mixture together until it forms a paste and then wrap it in a thin porous cloth. Spread a thin layer of Aloe Vera on the affected skin and then place the poultice over the area, then wrap or tape it in place.

Turmeric Poultice

Turmeric is a good **anti-fungal, anti-inflammatory** and **anti-microbial**. A Turmeric poultice is used on **Boils, Infections, Skin problems** as well as **Carpel-Tunnel Syndrome**, mostly due to Turmeric's **strong "drawing" properties**.

Recipe for Turmeric Poultice:

Add 2-3 drops of a vegetable oil (Olive Oil?) to 2-tbs. of Turmeric and blend well. Wrap the mixture in a thin sterile cloth and apply to the affected area. Wrap or tape the poultice to hold it in place.

As you can see the list of possible ingredients for Poultices is very long, and those listed here are just a few of the possibilities.

 Obviously, once you see the health applications of other Herbs and plants you can see that the use of combinations of these and even Essential Oils to make a Poultice that meets your specific needs is possible.

Even prepared Tinctures and Infusions work well as a part of Poultices.

How to Make a TINCTURE

Tinctures are concentrated extracts made from combinations of herbs or plants.

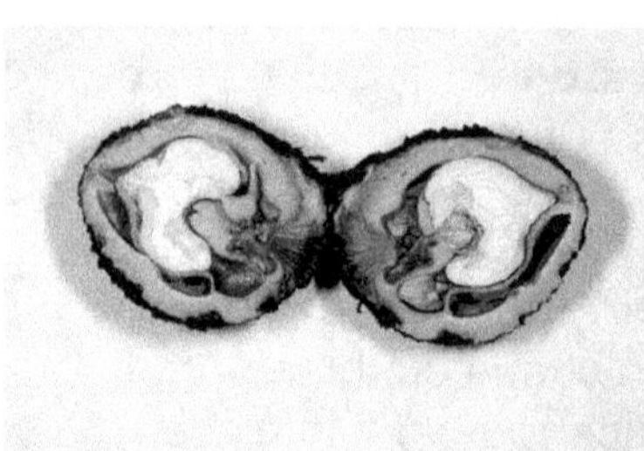

The particular parts of the plants used are usually fibrous and have to be chopped and mashed to facilitate the extraction of the essential oils when soaked in alcohols, usually Vodka.

Tinctures keep the extracted plant's ingredients stable and they usually act quickly when used as a health treatment.

BLACK WALNUT Tincture

A Black Walnut Tincture is used primarily for **skin diseases like; Athlete's foot, eczema, ringworm, impetigo, Ringworm and jock itch** to name a few. The tincture, which by the way will stain the skin, is used externally for these ailments.

Some people will use water rather than Vodka to make this tincture.

Even though the water-based tincture is not a true tincture, it is still used the same way, and it will not sting as bad as the true Vodka

Note that when you are treating a skin disease you should make sure that the person being treated drinks plenty of water.

based version.

Recipe for Black Walnut Hull Tincture, Alcohol based.

Wearing gloves, gather fallen Black Walnut nuts, that are green or green and brown, from the ground under the Walnut tree.
1. Remove the soft outer husks and place them into a quart jar.
2.   Cover the husks with a cheap Vodka or grain alcohol.
3.   Be sure to cover the Husks totally.
4.   Seal the jar and allow it to sit for about 1 week.
5.   Open the jar and strain the mixture through a cloth and into another clean jar.

6. Add water to the liquid, in a 50-50 mixture and seal the jar.
7. You now have enough Black Walnut Tincture
8. The Tincture will last for 6-10 months.
9. Keep the jar sealed and store it in the fridge or a cool place.

CANNABIS Tincture

Marijuana is very harsh to many people who are prescribed medical Marijuana. Considering most people do not smoke at all just learning to smoke is a hard thing for a person who is already sick

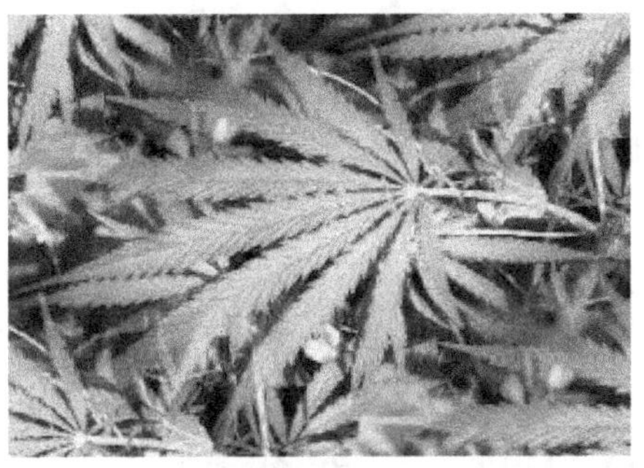

On top of that, many people who use **Medical Marijuana**, do not like having the odor of Marijuana smoke in their homes any more than they do having regular cigarette smoke smelling things up.

To resolve this issue, many doctors are prescribing the use of a **Cannabis Tincture** in your favorite Herbal Tea or under the tongue. It will provide the same relief for the ill person and not be as hard to take or have the odor.

Smoking Cannabis actually puts the active ingredients into the lungs and directly into the blood stream. Taking it orally, in a tea and through the stomach can require as much as ten times the amount of Cannabis for the same medicinal effect.

Use a tincture and get the same power of the drug by placing a couple of drops under the tongue and holding it there for several minutes before you swallow. This procedure, similar to smoking it, puts the active ingredients directly into the blood stream via the veins under the tongue.

Recipe for CANNABIS TINCTURE:
1. Finely grind your Cannabis plant pieces in a blender.
2. Fill a glass quart jar about ¾ full with your ground Marijuana.
3. Then cover the Marijuana completely with a high alcohol content Vodka.
4. Then, stir the mixture together well, even shaking it heartily, making sure that the Vodka soaks into every part of the Marijuana.
5. Seal the mixture in an Amber colored jar and shake it vigorously twice a day for at least two weeks or until the leaves have lost their green color.

6. Strain the liquid into a medicine dropper bottle for immediate use and reseal the large jar to age for future use.
7. The liquid will be a deep green color and will easily stain anything it gets on.

Tincture Dosage:

The tincture is strong and will burn, so, if it is used under the tongue mix the tincture with water or with a flavored syrup, in the ratio of 2-drops tincture to 1-drop syrup before placing it under the tongue.

If used in an **Herbal Tea**, the same thing applies, but it will need to be stronger when taken orally.

Mix from a half to a full dropper of tincture into the tea. If it's a bitter, add a flavoring. Cool the Tea a little before mixing flavorings with it, as heat will dissipate some of the power of the tincture.

Repeat the dosage as often as necessary.

EUCHINACEA Tincture

Echinacea Tincture is good for treating: **Colds, Chicken Pox, Influenza, Infections, Shingles Toothaches and even Urinary Tract Infections**.

Recipe for **EUCHINACEA Tincture:**

To make this tincture use the following process:
1- Cut up and place either fresh or dried Echinacea roots into a jar. Cover the roots with Vodka.
2- Seal the jar and allow it to sit for at least 30 days.
3- Every 2 or 3 days shake the bottle to accelerate the blending.
4- Strain the liquid from the mixture and place it into a sealable amber-colored bottle for use.

When using the tincture be sure to use regular dosages, and take it often, to fight the specific health problem.

CLEAN AIR in your HOME

We all want to breath fresh air in our homes. Air that is rich in oxygen and with as low as possible levels of other often toxic chemicals is not only healthier, but higher levels will stimulate your body and your mind to be more active. So you need to make sure you have done the things you can that will improve your home's air quality.

OPEN the WINDOWS - At certain times of the year, usually in the Spring, you should open your windows and allow the outside air into the house to freshen the inside air and eliminate those, so typical, stale odors from a Winter of keeping your house sealed from the elements. Doing this is an effective way to get rid of many of those toxins that have built up inside your house.

CLEAN AIR FILTERS – This is one of the things we can all do in our homes, **change the air filters** in our heating/cooling systems regularly. But, the majority of us will let this task go until either there is a problem, or we accidentally remember. And, when we do change the filter, it will be clogged with dust, pollen and dirt. The more often we do change these filters, the better the air in our home will be.

There are a few other thing you can do, such as use natural air fresheners, to detoxify the air in your home

HOUSE PLANTS as AIR FILTERS - By placing green leafy plants strategically around your home the air in your house will be freshened naturally.

These plants will continually absorb carbon dioxide and generate oxygen for you to breath.

Additionally, they will absorb such chemicals in the air as; **Benzene, formaldehyde**, and **trichloroethylene**.

According to **NASA, the top House Plants** to have for fresher air are;

- English Ivy, Spider Plant, Golden Pothos (or Devil's Ivy), Peace Lily, Chinese Evergreen, Bamboo Palm (or Reed Palm), Snake Plant (or Mother-in-law's Tongue), Heartleaf Philodendron, Selloum Philodendron, Elephant Ear Philodendron, Red-edged Dracaena, Cornstalk Dracaena, Janet Craig Dracaena, Warneck Dracaena, Weeping Fig, Gerbera daisy (or Barberton daisy), Pot Mum (or Florist's Chrysanthemum, Rubber plant.

<u>AROMATICS</u> - You can also use certain **Essential Oils** that are popular for their scents, such as Lavender, Mint, and others.

By placing these Oils in decorative bowls or just placing a few drops onto some Potpourri mixture, your air will be pleasingly freshened for days before needing to be refreshed.

These Oils are natural and not only provide a fresh scent and are a great source of aromatherapy, but you get to select the specific scent that suites your tastes.

HOME HEALTH TIPS for the SURVIVALIST

There are many things a person can do to improve or manage their Health or even treat certain physical problems without having to use those, oh so convenient and expensive, products sold in drugstores, supermarkets and on line on the web.

Home Treatments for Common Health problems

The following Tips and Treatments are recommended for the average person to consider implementing when they have the listed **Common Health problems**.

 Most of these treatments are themselves the same simple remedies used for centuries by our ancestor's for successfully treating these common problems.

It is also most likely that these treatments will also save them money on Doctor visits and prescription drugs, often utilizing items you already have in their home, garden or nearby woodlands.

ACNE

Acne is a skin disease that is a combination of areas of redness, blackheads and pimples. There are a number of home remedies that can work for some people and here are a few:

Treatment-1 – Mix 2-tbs. of **Healing Earth** (found in Health stores) with 2-tbs. of water to make a paste and apply it as a skin mask. Leave it on for 30 minutes and then wash off. Repeat 3-4 times a week.

Treatment-2 – Mix 2-tbs. of **Yogurt** with 1-tbs. of **Honey** to make a paste. Apply the paste to the face and leave it on for 30-minutes before washing it off. Repeat 2-3 times a week.

Treatment-3 – Mix 1-drop of **Tea Tree Oil** with 4 drops of water and apply it to any blackheads or pimples with a cotton ball. Wait 5-10 minutes and then wash the skin well.

ARTHRITIC PAIN

Arthritic Pain is generally a result of aging and worn joints in the body and these pains can be excruciating at times. There is no actual cure for worn out bodies but there are things that can be taken to ease the pains that are not prescription drugs.

Tart Cherry - Tart Cherries are very high in **antioxidants** and **beta-carotene**. Eating the Cherries, or more conveniently, drinking the popular Tart Cherry Juice works well in relieving a **sore throat, laryngitis**, and **stomach problems** and in reducing **Arthritic Pain** and **Gout**.

Tart Cherries also contain **melatonin** that makes it a good **natural sleep aid**.

Glucosamine – Glucosamine is another popular natural substance used successfully by many people to ease the pain of **osteoarthritis**.

It is actually made from the exoskeletons of crustaceans and certain fungi. Glucosamine is not a drug and is actually classified as a dietary supplement.

BURNS and SCALDS

There are a number of home remedies for Burns and Scalds.

First of all there are several levels of burns that one can suffer from and each is treated differently.

A **first-degree** burn, or superficial burn is one that involves only the outer layer of skin and even though a first-degree burn may be painful, it is easily treated.

A **second-degree** burn on the other hand is a burn to the deeper layers of flesh and often results in a blister and can often develop in to infections. This type of burn is more serious that a first-degree burn but it is still relatively easy to treat.

Then there is a **third-degree** burn which includes damage to the full thickness of the flesh. This is the most serious type of burn to treat and often entails the need for skin surgery.

 Below are a few different treatments to select from for first and second degree burns.

Cornstarch Paste Compress

Cornstarch Paste works very well to sooth most burns to the skin and making a Cornstarch Paste Compress is relatively simple.

RECIPE: First, slowly add warm water to 1-cup of Cornstarch until it reaches the consistency of a thick paste. Then fold the paste into a clean damp cloth and place the resultant compress over the burn area.

Aloe Vera

When Aloe Vera is used on burns it not only gives a cooling sensation to the skin but it also acts as a moisturizer and aids in skin rejuvenation if applied quickly and then reapplied every few hours right after the burn occurs.

Lavender Oil

Apply 4 to 8 drops of lavender oil onto a thin cloth and apply the oily side to the burn. Leave the compress on the burn for a couple of hours.

Sauerkraut

Crush fresh Sauerkraut (fermented Cabbage, add a few drops of a vegetable oil (Olive Oil?) and fold the mixture into a cloth. Apply the oily side of the cloth to the burn area and leave for several hours.

St. John's Wort

Make a compress by dabbing a small amount of St. John's Wort onto a cotton cloth and fold it on itself several times. Hold this compress, oily side down, on the burn or scald for 30 minutes.

Butter – Warning:

Do not apply Butter to a Burn because it can encourage the growth of bacteria on the skin.

COLD PREVENTION

Gargle with Water - People who gargle regularly with warm water, will have fewer attacks of Colds and Respiratory Infections. Gargling regularly reduces bacteria and germs in the mouth and helps many people prevent contracting a Cold.

Reduce Physical Contact with Others – During the Cold season, avoid direct physical contact with others. It takes several days for cold symptoms to show after you're infected and physical contact is the leading cause.

Try to **avoid shaking hands** wherever possible. Try using the "Fist Bump" with your friends when possible as this allows the least skin contact with others. Or, just say, "I think I might have a Cold" to avoid embarrassment when a hand is offered to shake.

Avoid Public Places – When you are in public places, avoid touching things that can pass bacteria on to you. Some of the places and things that have the highest probability of being infected are those touched the most by the public.

Avoid; utensils on restaurant **buffet lines**, **magazines** in doctors offices and waiting rooms, public building **door handles** and especially **restroom door handles**. And of course, wash your hands often throughout the day.

COMMON COLD:

There are a number of plants and herbs that have been established as good tools for helping cure common colds. Below are a number of the more popular cures that you can try.

Garlic Soup: Garlic Soup is high in antioxidants and this simple soup made with fresh Garlic with a few other herbs is an excellent and popular treatment for the common cold.

RECIPE: Mince a dozen or so cloves of Garlic and add ½-tsp. of salt and any other healthy herbs, of your choice, for added flavor (or to suppress the Garlic flavor?).

Mix the ingredients together well, add the blend to 3-4 cups of chicken stock and then bring the mixture to a low boil.

Once it is at a boil, turn off the heat and allow the mixture to cool. Pour the mixture through a sieve and then drink at least one cup of the liquid 2-3 times a day for relief of your cold.

Ginger Tea:

The Ginger Root can be used to treat the common cold by making a Ginger Tea with the minced fresh root to drink to relax and heal.

Onion and Honey Syrup Paste: Make this paste to treat and help cure a common cold.

RECIPE: Place one large red onion and 1/2 cup of water into a blender and mix together well.

Let the mixture sit for around 12 hours and then strain the liquid from the mixture. Mix the liquid with 2 tbs. of Honey and then allow this to sit for 3-4 hours.

Take the resultant syrup one spoonful at a time to help cure a common cold.

Other Useful Plants and Herbs for the Common Cold: There are a number of other herbs and essential oils that can be useful to treat the common cold and the Flu.

Some of the most popular ones used around the world are;
Eucalyptus Oil, Lemon Juice, Licorice Root and Red Onions.

Always be sure to take care with any of these treatments and for
safety's sake avoid using them on small children.

COMPRESS

A Soothing Compress will often ease pains resulting from burns,
and other skin damage as well as muscle pains. There are several
popular compresses you can make from common ingredients.

When making and using a compress, always be sure to clean the
wound properly and be sure that any plants you might use have
been washed adequately.

Milk Compress- Mix cold water with milk (75-25 ratio) and make
sure that it is blended well, then soak a cloth in the mixture and
place on the affected area of the body.

Oatmeal Water Compress – Soak dry oatmeal (not flavored or
coated cereal) in warm water for a couple of hours. After it has had
time to be diluted, filter the mixture through a gauze material. Then
soak a cloth in the resultant oatmeal water and place it on the
problem area of the body.

COUGHs or SCRATCHY THROATs

Simple coughs or scratchy throats can be soothed by holding a
teaspoon of a 50-50 combination of Whiskey and Honey in your
mouth and then allowing it to slowly coat your throat.

Black Cherry Cough Syrup

Black Cherry Cough Syrup is a popular medicine that is easy to
make yourself that will provide relief
for a persistent cough.

It is a medicine that you should keep
around your home for use when
someone in the family develops a
serious cough.

The recipe you see here just uses
Cherry Tree bark and Vodka. It has a great and soothing cherry
flavor and actually works well to stop a cough.

RECIPE: To make this medicine, just fill a quart sized jar with cut up pieces of cherry tree bark and then top off the jar with a cheap strong Vodka making sure to cover all of the bark with the liquid.

Seal the jar and allow the mixture set for about a month, making sure to shake the mixture every 2-3 days. After the month is over, strain the mixture into a different sealable (amber colored) bottle and mix the liquid 50-50 with honey.

Shake the mixture well, seal the bottle and you now have your own homemade cough syrup that if kept sealed can have a shelf life of 3-4 months.

Black Cherry tree bark is available in health food stores if you do not own a tree of your own or if you do not have access to a tree for its bark.

DOSAGE: The proper dosage should be 1-tablespoon for an adult and 1-teaspoon for children that are at least three years old or older. Only give a couple of doses to a person a day. Have the patient hold the liquid in their mouth and slowly allow it to trickle down their throat over several minutes.

CUTS

Many Cuts that people get are not dangerous enough for stitches, but do require proper cleaning and treatment.

Turmeric Powder has strong **anti-bacterial** properties; which make it ideal for use on cuts.

RECIPE: Make a paste by combining ½-cup Turmeric Powder and a pinch of salt with rubbing alcohol to form a thick paste. Apply the paste to the external wounds.

Styptic Herbs – There are a number of natural herbs that have strong Styptic powers and if applied to a cut either directly or as part of a Poultice, the bleeding can be controlled quickly or even stopped. See the list of appropriate Poultices in this book.

DENTAL PAIN

Dental Pain can be excruciating and often there are more natural ways to control it temporarily rather than visiting a Dentist.

Cloves (and Clove Oil)

Cloves and Clove Oil both have a number of natural medicinal applications including the fact that it has been used for centuries as a dental anesthetic (it numbs parts of the mouth on contact) and at the same time it helps reduce fevers.

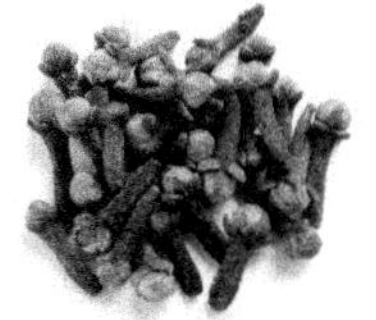

For temporary relief of toothache pain simply place a little **Clove Oil** onto a cotton swab and hold it on the pain filled area of gum or the tooth.

Clove Oil can also help expel certain parasitic worms from the gastro-intestinal tract, and it is a good mosquito repellant.

OIL PULLING:

Sesame Seed Oil is high in antioxidants, Omega-3 fatty acids and polyunsaturated fats as well as being a good source of Vitamins A, B, and E.

> **CAUTION**: Sesame Oil is toxic to some people and can cause allergic reactions, so while holding it in your mouth, do not swallow any of the liquid or allow any to trickle down your throat.

The process called Oil Pulling is popular in India for relieving tooth pains and tightening the gums. Oil Pulling is also very effective in removing bacteria from the mouth.

Follow this procedure;
1. Use 1-tbs of Sesame Seed Oil (or Gingelly Oil) and place it in the mouth.
2. Swish it around for 15-20 minutes before spitting the liquid out.
3. The liquid should be a milky color when you spit it out. (If not, you did not swish it around long enough.).
4. Rinse the mouth thoroughly with warm water and then brush your teeth thoroughly.
5. Drink a couple of glasses of water afterward to dilute any of the liquid you may have inadvertently swallowed.
6. Repeat this process once a day, in the morning until the pain has gone away.

This process works for mouth pains and if you use this same

> **CAUTION**: Do not allow children to perform this process, as they may not be able to do it properly. Teens or small adults can use only 1-tsp. for the process.

process using Coconut Oil, it will slowly remove tooth stains giving you whiter teeth.

Sunflower Oil, although not as effective, can also be used for Oil Pulling and the reduction of dental pain.

EAR INFECTIONS

If you suspect you have an Ear Infection, or your ears are stopped up or itching, it is possible to treat this problem at home.

Brewer's Yeast: One common treatment for ear infections is the use of Brewer's Yeast. By taking it a dietary supplement brewer's yeast has been found to be useful for managing a number of health problems including; **Acne, Boils, Diarrhea** and even reducing **Blood Sugar** levels.

Warning: Brewer's Yeast can help cure an ear infection for most people, but some people are allergic to yeasts and you should avoid using brewer's yeast if you are allergic.

OLIVE OIL has been used to treat ear infections successfully for centuries. Use only the best olive oils such as either **EVOO** (Extra Virgin Olive Oil) or first-cold pressed versions.

Process:
1. Apply only one or two drops into the infected ear.
2. After a minute or two, allow the oil to drain naturally from the ear.
3. Repeat the process to the infected ear several times a day to get rid of the infection.

EYES & EYELIDS, ITCHY, RED, CRUSTY

If you often have itchy red eyelids, this is often called Blepharitis, which a common ailment in older adults.

One way to ease this problem is to mix a 50/50 solution of a mild baby shampoo and warm water. Gently rub this on eyelids (not the eyes) and it will help remove bacteria and oils. And, it will not sting your eyes.

The old trick of placing Cucumber slices on the eyelids will reduce the swelling but it will also help with red eyes.

Red Eyes

If you have Red Eyes, you must first stop rubbing them. Rubbing red irritated eyes will only irritate them more. Using a compress made with **Daisy buds** that have been soaked in warm water, or **Eyebright**, placed lightly over closed eyes will relieve the pain.

EYELIDS, Swollen

Swollen Eyelids are typically a result of a buildup of fluid in the tissue of the eyelid itself and usually a cold compress will reduce this swelling. Some other treatments are:

Cure-1 – Apply slice of Cucumber to the eyelids for 10-minutes.

Cure-2 – Place natural Yogurt onto a damps cloth to make a compress and place this onto the eyelids for 10-15 minutes.

FISH OIL

Fish Oil contains the **Omega-3 fatty acids, EPA** (*eicosapentaenoic acid)* and **DHA** (docosahexaenoic acid) that are both known to help **reduce inflammation** in the human body.

Eating fatty cold-water fish such a Salmon provides some of these acids. The oil is usually taken in the form of **Fish Oil** capsules.

Although it is still considered a healthy addition to most people's supplement lists, the use of Fish oil for lowering Cholesterol has been disputed recently by several respected scientific studies.

FOOD POISONING Symptoms

Food Poisoning happens more often than it should and it usually occurs from eating foods that are not clean or sanitary. The most common sources are improperly washed vegetables and fruits.

Food Poisoning will generally **occur within two to six hours of eating** unclean foods, and typical symptoms are **nausea, diarrhea, stomach cramps, overall weakness, along with fever, chills** and **headaches.**

There are a number of **germs that can cause food poisoning**, including; Campylobacter enteritis, Cholera, E.coli enteritis, Fish poisoning, Staphylococcus aureus, Salmonella and Shigella

Recovering: To recover quickly, you need to; manage your diarrhea, control your nausea and vomiting and get plenty of rest.

Dehydration: Take care, especially if you are **vomiting**, to drink plenty of fluids in order to avoid dehydration. Lost Fluids and electrolytes is the most dangerous problem that results from food poisoning and you need to push fluids through your body in order for it to recover quickly.

GLUCOSAMINE and Pain

Glucosamine is not a drug. In fact it is a natural chemical that is found in the shells of crustaceans as well as in the bone marrow of some animals.

Glucosamine Sulfate is available, over the counter, and has been proven to act as an **anti-inflammatory**.

It is very popular in treating **osteoarthritis** for must adult sufferers.

GOUT

Gout is the **inflammation of joints caused by high uric acid levels in the body**. The uric acid tends to settle into the body's extremities, typically at night while the person is asleep.

This uric acid often solidifies into grains similar to sand in the joints of the extremities and this is what causes the extreme pain.

Tart Cherry Juice is high in **antioxidants** and is also rich in potassium among other nutrients.

Drinking a teaspoon of tart cherry Juice daily will often aid in reducing the level of uric acid in the body and thus help prevent gout attacks.

> Tart Cherry Juice is also good for treating Insomnia due to its relatively high content of melatonin.

Steroids, such as prescription prednisone are anti-inflammatories and a daily regiment taken for one to 1-1/2 weeks can reduce the inflammation and ease the symptoms of gout.

Prescription non-steroid drugs such as Colchicine will temporarily reduce the inflammation.

DIET CONTROL: Losing Weight, exercising and eating low-acid foods will help reduce the occurrence and severity of Gout attacks for most people.

Avoid red meat, Seafood and foods that contain Yeasts.

DRINK FLUIDS: Drink plenty of fluids daily to help lower the Uric Acid level in the body and thus avoid Gout attacks.

HAIR GROWTH Stimulant

If you want to potentially stimulate hair growth, use those leftover cucumber peels. They are beneficial because they contain silica, which strengthens collagen, which, in turn, has been proven to help accelerate hair growth in some people.

Place the **cucumber peels** in a blender along with just enough oil (Olive Oil) to mince the peels into a paste.

Take the resultant mixture and rub it onto the scalp for a couple of hours while relaxing at home. Then, of course, wash the mixture from your hair and repeat again the next day.

HONEY and its uses

Honey is, as we all know, produced by Honey Bees and has been used by humans for thousands of years. In addition to its wonderful sweet flavor, it is a **natural anti-bacterial** and **antiseptic**.

It has been used to treat **Allergies, Burns, Colds, Coughs, Gastric Ulcers, Wounds**, and more.

RECIPE: A popular recipe is to mix 2-tbs. of Honey with 1-tsp. of lemon juice in a cup of hot water and drink the mixture. Add a little cinnamon if you like to strengthen the power of the cure as well as for the flavor.

CAUTION: Honey should not be given to babies.

NOTE: To rehydrate dried up Honey, simply add some water to the container and allow the mixture to sit, shaking it occasionally, until it reforms into its liquid form.

HIGH BLOOD PRESSURE

Eventually, ending up with High Blood Pressure is almost a "right of passage" as people in this world of ours mature and start to live the modern lifestyle; one of high stress and poor eating habits.

Well, changing ones job or making radical changes to your lifestyle can be hard for many of us to accomplish, but there are a number of things that you can do to improve your chances of lowering your blood pressure.

Listed here are a few of the more natural things that we can all do to help reduce our blood pressure;

Drink less Alcohol.

Alcohol consumption can contribute to a person having higher blood pressure, so if you want to lower your BP, reduce your drink consumption to two drinks or less a day.

Drink less Milk products.

Save milk-based foods such as desserts and such as an occasional treat and not a part of your regular diet.

Eat more Garlic.

Garlic is a great natural food that you can eat that is known for its ability to help control High Blood Pressure as well as High Cholesterol. So, pull out your recipe book and cook more dishes with Garlic in them.

Yogurt is a great food that is not only nutritious but provides a number of health benefits for the regular consumer. I recommend purchasing the "Greek-style" yogurts because they are thicker with less water added to them. But watch out for dangers from some of the additives the manufacturers might slip in on you; even the supposedly safe fruits, etc.

Exercise more.

Get up and start some kind of regular exercise program that will help keep your heart healthy and will probably lower your BP. It is now recommended that walking three or more times a week for 20-30 minutes will make a difference in your hearts health; and can lower your BP.

Get enough Sleep.

Sleep is very important to your health and too many people do not get enough, which can contribute to higher blood pressure. Plan ahead and allow yourself enough time each night for adequate rest.

Plan the two or so hours before you go to bed for restful situations that will allow you to go to bed ready to sleep. Do not drink caffeine drinks, do not watch scary or high action TV shows, and go to bed in a room that is comfortable and quiet as all of these can contribute to a better nights sleep.

Reduce Stress.

Tests have shown that one of the easiest ways to lower your BP is to make an effort to reduce the day-to-day stress in your life. Stressful situations can raise your BP dramatically. Take those regularly occurring situations and find a way to manage them calmly. Over time, this will lower those instances of high BP caused by stress.

HOUSE SPIDERS and TREATMENTS

There are three major varieties of venomous spider that can be found in the US. These poisonous pests are; the Black Widow Spider, the Brown Recluse Spider and the Hobo Spider.

BLACK WIDOW SPIDER:

The female Black Widow spider known for its unique markings is much more poisonous than the male. They are found in homes because they prefer a warm environment.

The Black Widow has several natural enemies such as; the blue mud dauber and the spider wasp.

> **NOTE:** Actually when you see any spider with a large abdomen it should be avoided as it could be poisonous.

BROWN RECLUSE SPIDER:

The Brown Recluse spider is poisonous but it prefers to stay hidden in a quiet and warm environment for nesting. It is brown and has a fiddle shaped body and only six eyes as opposed to the normal eight. They have no known natural predator.

HOBO SPIDER:

The poisonous Hobo spider looks a lot like the Brown Recluse but has a mottled back coloring and a herringbone pattern on its abdomen. It has several natural enemies including; the Jumping Spider, the Crab Spider, and the Wolf Spider.

Spider Bite SYMPTOMS: According to the CDC, there are a number of symptoms that come with a venomous spider bite and they include; Itching or Rash, pain radiating from the site, muscle pain or cramps, skin a reddish or purple color, sweating, difficulty breathing, headache, nausea, vomiting, chills, and high blood pressure.

SPIDER VENOM TREATMENTS: Although most spider bites are not deadly to adults, they can be so for children. Take a picture of the spider for later confirmation, wash the site with soap and water, keep the limb elevated, take regular pain relievers, and make sure the site does not become infected.

You should see a physician immediately if you begin to have severe pain, abdominal cramping or a growing ulcer at the bite site.

INFUSED OILS

Infused Oils have been used for thousands of years for healing numerous health problems.

RECIPE: The process for making an infused oil of your favorite herb is relatively simple.

1. Place the fresh herbs you wish to infuse in a pan and add enough oil to cover them totally (typically, Almond oil, Coconut oil or Olive oil).
2. Cover and heat the mixture in an oven at a temperature of 115F to 200F until the herbs have become crispy, which should take from 2-4 hours.
3. Once the herbal material is crispy, (this is an indication that the process is done) the herbal oils have been extracted from the solids.
4. Separate the liquid from the solids with a sieve.
5. Bottle the liquid in a sterilized amber or colored, sealable jar.

The Oil is ready to be used as an ointment. The liquid can be preserved to last longer by adding one Vitamin E capsule to the liquid before sealing the jar.

Some popular infused oils that you can make are:

Calendula makes a good **antiseptic, anti-fungal** and **wound healing ointment**.

Comfrey is actually a good **soothing emollient** and an ointment made from Comfrey helps treat **sore muscles and joints** and is even purported to **help heal broken bones**.

Plantain, which grows wild, is a good **astringent, anti-viral, anti-inflammatory** and **anti-microbial**. The ointment is **good for treating rashes,** even **diaper rash** on babies.

St. John's Wort, which grows wild around the world, acts as a **sedative** and as an **anti-inflammatory**.

Slippery Elm Bark provides soothing **relief to burns** and **wounds** and **promotes healing**.

Yarrow, also known as **Soldier's Woundwort** is an **astringent** and an **anti-inflammatory** which has been used for centuries to treat **bleeding wounds, cuts** and abrasions by slowing the blood flow, and promoting healing.

These are but a few of the many other herbs can also be used in making great and useful ointments for treating common ailments and health problems.

Make a Salve: Almost all **Infused Oils can be made into salves** by placing them into a small pan and adding beeswax. Heat the combination over a low heat until the wax melts and combines with the ointment. Place the salve in a sealable large-mouth jar for future use.

INSECT BITES or STINGS

Some people are allergic to insect bites or stings much more than others and if you are one of these people you should seek medical attention immediately when attacked.

 On the other hand, if you do not have such allergies, for most people the pain of insect bites and stings can be handled with some simple home remedies.

Cold Compress: The pain of an insect bite can often be eased by applying a cold compress or just by running cold water over the site.

Clean the Area: You should clean the area of a sting with soap and water and then you can place fresh lemon or onion directly onto the site; the acid will neutralize the pain.

Baking Soda Paste: A paste made of baking soda and water will also ease the pain of insect bites and stings.

Poultices: To treat more serious Insect bites and avoid infections try some of the poultices listed in this book.

TICK BITES:

Ticks can be more than just a physical nuisance when you get one on your body.

Seasonally, when you are out and walking under trees, especially certain trees such as Pines and such, you run the risk of a Tick dropping from the tree and onto your body.

Once they are on you, they will crawl to a good spot on you and bite into the skin. Once they are attached, they begin the process of sucking your blood.

The real problems with Ticks is not just the bite, but the numerous diseases they can be carrying that could infect you, such as Lymes Disease for one.

The most important thing to do when you come inside is to check your body thoroughly for Ticks. If you find one, you need to remove it immediately.

How to remove a Tick:

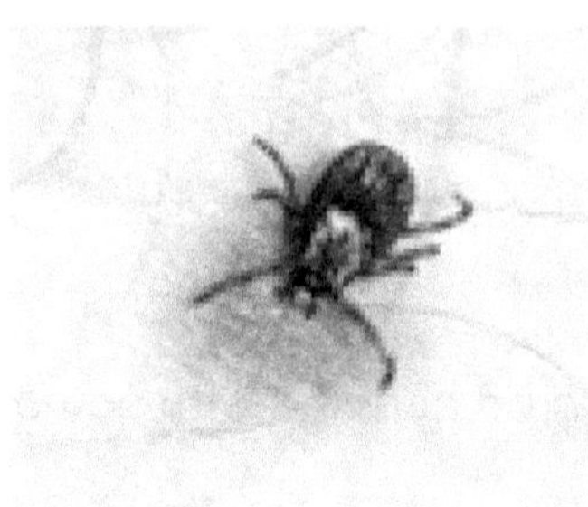

According to the CDC, the best way to remove a Tick from the skin is to use a pair of tweezers, grasp the body and gently pull upwards.

Do not twist the body or pull too hard. The Tick should let go after a few seconds.

If the body pulls away from the head, use the tweezers to remove the head.

Once the Tick is removed, clean the area of the skin with alcohol as well as your hands. Or clean with Iodine.

DO NOT use the old folklore remedies and coat the Tick and skin with such things as gels or nail polish to get it to die or fall off. The Tick needs to be removed immediately to avoid infections, etc.

MOSQUITO MANAGEMENT

Damned Mosquitos! How often have you heard this or something similar while outside and enjoying the wonders of nature?

People spend millions of dollars annually, in vain efforts to keep Mosquitos from dining on their blood. Below are a few things that you can do to temporarily stop or at least reduce the number of mosquito bites that you might suffer.

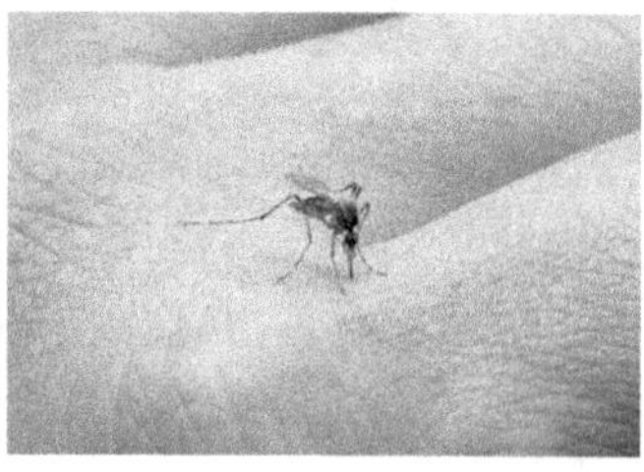

But remember that factors such as the temperature, level of sweating and exposure to water can vary the effectiveness of the repellant.

Prevention-1 – Cover up. That's right cover up. The more of your flesh that is covered up, the less area there is for a mosquito to land on and dine.

Prevention-2 – The repellant **OLE (Oil of Lemon Eucalyptus)** is an excellent natural mosquito repellant that is made form the distillation of the OLE component from the leaves of the Lemon Eucalyptus tree.

It is approved by the EPA for use on humans. It protects skin for up to 6-hours and should not be used on children younger than three years old, or older if small in stature for their age.

Prevention-3 – The repellant **Catnip Oil** is made through the distillation of the oil from the catnip plant itself. Its active component is Nepetalactone which is a strong mosquito repellant that can last for up to 15-hours. The more of the active ingredient in the spray, the longer it is effective, so follow the instruction.

Prevention-4 – **Citronella Oil** can repel mosquitos but it must be reapplied at least every hour to continue its effectiveness.

The **best mosquito control** that has proven most effective is to concentrate on controlling the environment where they prefer to produce and lay their larvae. No newly hatching mosquitos means no mosquito bites.

By the way, only the female Mosquito bites and draws blood, not the male.

LOW IRON

Having Low Iron levels in your body can lead to numerous ailments including; tiredness, lethargy, weakness, inflamed tongue, a weak immune system, among others.

Often, just eating adequate quantities of the right **iron-rich foods** can cure this illness.

Some foods that are rich in Iron are; **Red Meats, Mushrooms, dark green leafy vegetables, Turnip Greens, Kale, Spinach, Swiss Chard, Lentils, Parsley, Broccoli, Chick Peas (Garbanzo Beans)** and **Beans in general**, just to name a few.

MUSCLE CRAMPS, Foot and Leg

Foot and Leg Cramps are extremely painful for those who suffer this complaint.

Often the pain of a foot cramp can be eased simply by standing up and then walking on the afflicted foot. A leg cramp can also be eased by purposely stretching the cramping leg muscle, as well.

Epsom Salt baths can ease the pain of Foot and Leg Cramps.

Adequate levels of the two minerals Calcium and Magnesium are both necessary to a properly functioning body. So some repeat sufferers should take supplement pills for these minerals.

Muscle Cramps are most often caused by **Magnesium deficiencies** in the body. Or rather a deficiency relative to amount of Calcium consumed. To avoid Foot and Leg Cramps, there must be a balance of these two Minerals in the body with the person

> **NOTE:** Calcium is stored in the body while Magnesium is excreted; so one sign of consuming too much Magnesium is Diarrhea.

consuming neither too much nor too little of either one.

If a person has these cramps often then they need to simply change their diet by adding such foods as; beans, dark green leafy vegetables, nuts, seeds and whole grains to increase the body's levels of Magnesium.

PAIN RELIEF & Muscle Relaxers

Herbs have been used for thousands of years for pain relief and as muscle relaxers.

The ones listed below are some of the most popular. Obviously, you should always consult your physician before taking any herbal remedy either alone or with a prescribed drug.

Most Herbs work best when they are combined with other supportive Herbs so when shopping, you will often find these Herbs in a mixture with others.

Arnica is a species of flowering plant, often found in North America that contains a chemical known as *helenalin*.

This ingredient acts as an **anti-inflammatory** and **antibiotic**. It is even used to aid in the **treatment of tumors** as well as being a popular treatment for muscle pain.

WARNING: It should be used with caution because overdosing can cause such problems as **gastroenteritis** and even **internal bleeding**.

Boswellia is a species of tree whose bark contains a chemical with strong **anti-inflammatory** properties.

It is often used to **treat depression, fevers, rheumatism** and even **gastro-intestinal problems**.

Cayenne Pepper provides effective pain relief when used topically as a poultice.

Chamomile is an herb known for thousands of years as a good **muscle relaxer** and is often used in conjunction with other Herbs for maximum effect.

Devil's Claw is a good **anti-inflammatory** that is often used to relieve pain.

Horsetail provides strong pain relief that should be used with caution.

Kava Root is often used for pain relief.

Licorice is an Herb that is used for its **anti-inflammatory** properties that are similar to those of steroids.

Passiflora is often used as a muscle relaxer.

Red Onions are rich in the flavonoid, quereetin, which is used to improve **gastro-intestinal health**.

Also, Red Onions are a **strong anti-inflammatory** useful for treating problems with the throat, and blood vessels as well as the bones.

Valerian is an herb that is a strong **anti-inflammatory** that relieves pain and helps relax muscles. It can also help induce sleep.

White Willow Tree Bark contains the **natural painkiller** Salicin; which is **similar to Aspirin**. It has worked well for thousands of years to **treat fevers and pains**.

NUTRITIONAL Balance is very important to minimize body pains. To this end, you should always make sure that your body is getting enough of these important nutrients: Calcium, Magnesium, Potassium, Silica and Vitamin C.

PINK EYE

Pink Eye is the common name for **Conjunctivitis** that is actually a **highly contagious infection of the eyes**. If you have this problem, you should see a Doctor right away. A person can get irritated eyes that will appear red from such things as exposure to smoke, chlorinated water or other irritants in the air.

To treat irritated eyes, keep them clean by **cleaning the eyelids** with water on something soft such as a cotton ball. Clean them several times a day.

You can use the herb, **Eyebright** to give your eyes an **eye bath**.

This is done by chopping the herb finely and placing 1-2 tsp. into a cup of boiling water.

Once the water mixture it is lukewarm, place the wet herb onto a sterile soft cloth and place it over the closed eyes for up to 10-minutes. This can be repeated 2-3 times a day.

PLANTAR WARTS

Plantar warts are usually removed by doctors using laser or surgical techniques. Their methods are not only painful but the surgery does not guarantee that the warts will not grow back.

On the other hand there is a natural way to kill Plantar Warts using **White Thyme Oil** (Red Thyme Oil is not as strong a product).

PROCESS:
1. Soak the foot with the Plantar Wart in hot water to soften the skin.
2. Dry the site of the wart and apply several drops of Thyme Oil (5-6 undiluted) directly to the wart.
3. Allow the oil to soak into the wart and skin and then dry it off.
4. Check the wart the next day and the skin will have turned black (the skin will be dead).
5. Use a pumice stone to remove the dead skin.
6. Repeat the steps above every other day for a month or so, or until all of the Plantar Wart is gone.

POISON IVY

Poison Ivy is a vine-like plant with dark green glossy leaves that are

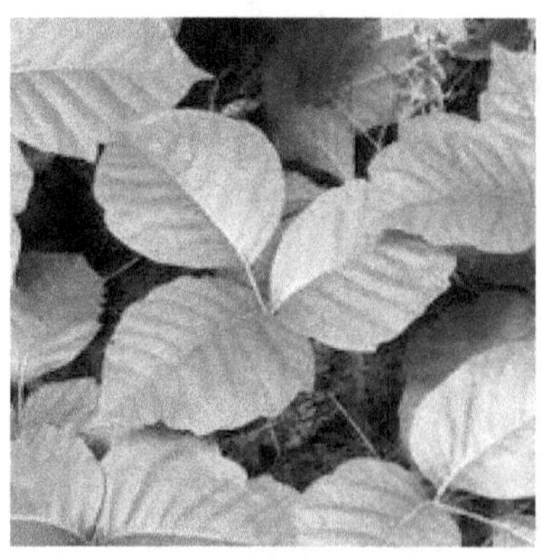

grouped in threes. The leaves, stalks, flowers and fruits of Poison Ivy all contain a yellowish oil called that affects people who are allergic to it with a rash that is hard to get rid of.

 The rash quickly turns to blisters and if scratched the rash and blisters will spread on the skin.

Treatments: Here are some popular home treatments that you can use to get rid of poison ivy:

WASH: Immediately wash yourself your clothes and everything that the plant may have touched.

Vitamin C: Drink lots of Vitamin-C based drinks.

Salt Water Bath: Soak the infected area in a salt-water bath to remove the oils immediately and regularly afterwards for relief of the itching.

Calamine Lotion: Using Calamine lotion on the rash to relieve the itch is very effective.

Avoid Scratching: Keep the area covered to reduce the chance of scratching, and do not scratch the area or open any blisters that do occur. Covering the area with a soft sterile cloth will not only reduce the chance of your scratching, but it will soak up any draining of the area or popped blisters.

Jewel Weed Poultice: Make a Jewel Weed Poultice and apply it to the infected skin.

There are probably a dozen or more home remedies for treating poison ivy but these seem to be considered the most effective.

If you end up with a severe case of poison ivy, or if it has not gone away after 10-days, you should contact your physician immediately to properly contain this common summer ailment.

SHOULDER SORENESS

A sore shoulder can have several causes, such as Osteoarthritis in which the pain is caused by one having the cartilage in the joint worn down or worn away.

The soreness is usually worst at night and for some people the joint may actually make a creaking sound from the bones rubbing on each other without the lubricating effect of cartilage. Often the joint will become swollen.

There is no cure for **Osteoarthritis**. Exercise that strengthens the surrounding muscles can provide some relief by stabilizing the joint but it will not cure the arthritis. Most doctors will simply recommend that you should modify your normal joint movements to shift the use of the worn area to areas that are nor worn out.

Witch Hazel Compress- Witch Hazel can often ease the pain from osteoarthritis.

Clean the fresh leaves of the plant well before using. Crush or chop the leaves well, into a mash. Place this or your purchased Witch Hazel extract into cold water and after it has set long enough to be diluted, soak a cloth in the solution and place it onto the body area.

Refresh your Compress in the solution every 30 minutes.

SKIN MOISTURIZER

Your skin is the largest organ of your body, and at times it can become dry which is actually not healthy. Normally, the human skin will generate its own oil protection, naturally but if the skin does become dry it can be revitalized through the regular use of any of a number of Essential Oils.

Two of the more popular Oils used as Skin Moisturizers are listed below:

Coconut Oil – The essential oil, Coconut Oil is the base for many commercial skin moisturizers. You can make your own by combining Coconut Oil any of several other oils of your own choice such as Olive Oil or Lavender, etc.

Lanolin - Lanolin is the natural oil in **Sheep's Wool** that provides them with protection against the weather. Lanolin is most like the oils on the skin of humans and makes a really good skin moisturizer.

SKIN PROBLEMS

Dry skin and other skin problems can often be controlled or even eliminated by using natural components such as certain Essential Oils and plant extracts.

Witch Hazel Extract - The extract made from North American variety of Witch Hazel is a natural astringent, and is used to treat such problems as **cracked skin, eczema, ingrown nails, psoriasis, varicose veins** and **hemorrhoids**. It is also used by some women to reduce swelling and to ease childbirth pains.

RECIPE: To make Witch Hazel extract you should soak fresh bark from the plant in Vodka, if you are going to use it internally. Or you can use Rubbing Alcohol if it is to be used externally. Dried bark will also work but it will have less of the oils that will be lost during the drying process.

Use only the bark from the part of the plant that is above ground in the area of the plant limbs. Do not use the roots!

Cover the mixture and allow it to soak for a couple of days before pouring it through a cloth or sieve to separate the liquid for later use.

SUNBURN

The Sun is a good source of Vitamin-D, but too much exposure to the Sun can result in serious sunburn. Even though it may seem OK, sunburn can often take months for a case of Sunburn to heal completely.

Sunburn **symptoms** include; **blistering, fever, itching, nausea and skin discoloration**.

For Sunburn prevention you should stay out of the direct Sun's Rays, especially during the peak sunshine period of the day that is typically from 10:00 AM to 3:00 PM.

You should wear long-sleeve shirts and broad brimmed hats when in the Sun and use a SPF-50 Sunscreen 20-30 minutes before going into the sunshine.

And, by eating foods that are high in anti-oxidants your body will have better tools to fight a burn.

SECONDARY SUNSHINE: You should always avoid being in direct sunlight for any extended period of time. Today, most doctors recommend only 20-30 minutes maximum time in the direct sunshine.

But, if you are going to be outside, especially on a vacation at the beach, sit under a good high-SPF umbrella. You will be surprised at the tan you can eventually get just from secondary sunshine, or the reflected sunshine.

And, take the same precautions as you would in direct sunshine because even this reflected sunshine can give you a serious burn, but at least it will take longer.

SUNBURN TREATMENTS: After the fact, relief from the pain and discomfort of a sunburn is the source of a lot of money for corporations who manufacture all types of ointments, salves and sprays. For a more natural approach to treatment, any of the following will work to relieve the symptoms and the pain:

Aloe Vera – Lightly rub the burned or sensitive area with Aloe Vera gel or the liquid from a leaf of the plant itself. In fact, Aloe Vera gel is such a versatile and effective tool that it is recommended that everyone have a potted Aloe Vera plant in their house for those time it is needed.

Milk Compress – Apply a soothing Milk Compress made of water and skim milk, oatmeal water, or Witch Hazel and water. These will ease the immediate pain and the milk and Witch Hazel both have anti-bacterial properties.

Cornstarch paste: Make this paste and apply it to the sunburned area for pain relief.

Keep HYDRATED by drinking at least 4-5 glasses of water a day. And yes, I said water, not alcohol-based drinks. Drinking adequate amounts of water helps speed up the healing process.

Apply OILS and Moisturizers that will act as soothing liquids to burned areas.

Rub the burn area with Yogurt to sooth the pain.

Eyelids - Apply moistened, used tea bags to burned eyelids to sooth and reduce any swelling and later apply a light layer of a moisturizing oil such as Olive oil.

INFECTED SKIN AREAS: If infection occurs, mix **Turmeric powder** with distilled water to make a paste and apply the paste to the infected area of the body.

TEETH WHITENING

In today's society, for some reason, it is desirable to not only have clean teeth and healthy gums, but to also have sparkling white teeth. Here are some things that you can do to whiten teeth without those dangerous chemicals that are on the market today.

BRUSH more often: It is a simple fact, the more often you brush your teeth, the more food particles you will remove, but the less stains will be left on your teeth, so brush several times a day for whiter teeth.

HYDROGEN PEROXIDE and BAKING SODA: The combination of these two common household items into a paste and using it once a week will remove tooth stains better than most commercial toothpastes used. Mix the two together until you have about ½-teaspoon of paste. Brush thoroughly with this paste and then rinse your mouth several time to remove any residue.

COCONUT OIL: Coconut Oil whitens teeth when used in the **Ayurvedic technique** also called **Oil Pulling**.

PROCESS: The process is a simple one. Place 1-tbs. of Coconut Oil in your mouth and hold it there. Then swish the oil around in your mouth for 15-20 minutes. Do not swallow the liquid.

Continue swishing the liquid for a total of up to 20-minutes and then spit the liquid out. Rinse your mouth out with water and then brush your teeth.

Perform this once a day, usually in the morning before you brush your teeth.

Over time, the Coconut Oil will draw the staining materials from your teeth and they will be whiter.

CALCIUM and your DIET: Make sure that your diet provides your body with the necessary levels of Calcium so you will have healthy teeth. Usually this can be achieved with the Calcium in most of the popular daily Multi-Vitamin pills.

USE a STRAW: If you like to drink beverages that are colored then you are probably adding more stains to your teeth than necessary. Make a habit of drinking all colored beverages with a straw as this will get the beverage past your teeth and avoid staining them.

VAPOR RUB, Homemade

A simple Vapor Rub, applied to the chest at night, can work wonders on someone, especially a child, who has sinus congestion.

The process to make your own Vapor Rub mixture is very easy and once made it will keep for months in its sealed container.

The basic rub is made with Beeswax and EVOO (Extra Virgin Olive Oil. While making it you will add a combination of several Essential Oils for their natural health benefits. These Oils are Eucalyptus, Peppermint and Rosemary. All of these can be found in health food stores or often in your local drug store.

RECIPE:
1. Place a glass bowl in a saucepan of water.
2. Place 1/4-cup of EVOO and 2-tsp of Beeswax in the bowl.
3. Heat until the beeswax melts and mix it together with the EVOO until well blended.
4. Remove the HOT bowl from the heat and set aside.
5. Begin adding the Essential Oils (15-drops-Eucalyptus, 25-drops-Peppermint, 12-drops-Rosemary) to the bowl while constantly blending into the mixture.
6. Pour the mixture into a sterilized, wide-mouth, sealable jar.

7.   Seal the jar and store in the fridge to allow the mixture to harden.

This mixture will last for 6-months to a year of kept sealed and in a cool place.

To Use: Do not apply or remove your Vapor Rub with your bare hands or you may end up with a cross-contamination problem. Use disposable gloves to rub the mixture into the skin of the back or chest and use throw-away sterile spatulas to remove the old mixture.

WARTS, MOLES and SKIN TAGS

Many of us have Moles, Warts and even skin tags on our bodies. Some of these are dangerous and all of them should be shown to your doctor for examination. On the other hand, many of these are deemed safe and not necessary to be removed. There are ways to get rid of these ugly thing son your skin, safely.

CASTOR OIL PASTE: Castor Oil is known for its ability to remove and dissolve tumors on the skin, among its other properties. Moles and Skin Tags can be removed with the application of a Castor Oil Paste.

Make the paste by mixing 2-3 drops of Castor Oil with 1-tsp. of baking soda. Place the paste on a thin cloth (or use a simple Band-Aid) and place it directly over the mole or skin tag.

Repeat the treatment twice a day until they drop off. The process can take up to 4-6-weeks but it does work.

Warts – This procedure also works on Warts for most people.

ESSENTIAL OILS and their BENEFITS

First of all, in case you didn't already know it, **Essential Oils** are not actually essential, per se, but are actually the basic (or essential) oil that can be extracted from a specific plant.

The plants that Essential Oils are extracted from have developed certain defensive mechanisms, over the eons of their evolution.

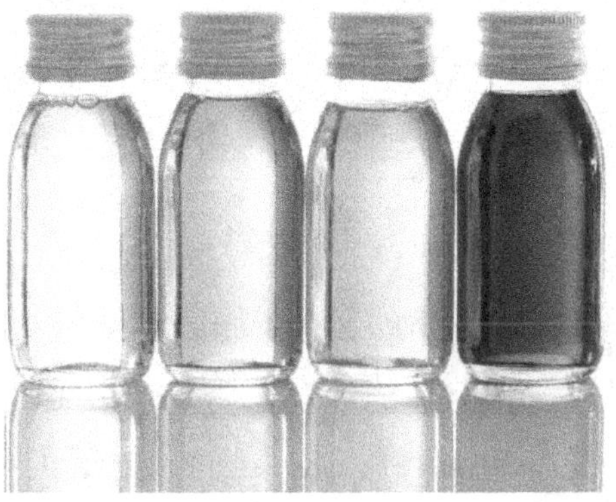

These defensive tools were developed by nature over time to protect the plants from diseases, weather, insects, and other particular environmental conditions that threatened the plants.

These defensive mechanisms are reflected in the unique chemicals that the plants produce naturally. Mankind, over thousands of years, has used these plants for treating particular health conditions in humans.

Essential Oils have been used as far back as the times of the Pharaohs and even further back in some civilizations. In fact, during those times in Egypt there were hundreds of popular essential oils recorded as being used.

They, were then, and still are, popular and even prized as aromatics, flavorings in food preparations, and of course special ingredients in many medical applications and even in embalming the dead.

Even today, there are numerous popular essential oils used in personal care products as well as medicinally to treat health problems.

Essential Oils are highly concentrated extractions from plants and flowers, so when you use them you will typically use small portions, whether for medicinal applications, aromatherapy or just to enjoy their fantastic fragrances.

Production Methods

Many herbs as well as numerous other plants are also used for their extractible chemicals to make essential oils and other natural condensed chemicals. These Herb oils are made by processing certain parts of a plant, typically its flowers, roots, bark or sometimes its stems, to break down their chemical components.

The majority of Essential Oils are produced by a distillation procedure using water but some are made using a technique referred to as Solvent Extraction.

The distillation process can be performed at home to make many of the popular essential oils used today.

NOTE: Some commercial Essential Oils do not have the strength of others that are processed properly. This is usually the case when, during the distillation process, the mixture is heated to a temperature above 180F.

The liquids are extracted and then condensed to give the essential oil itself. Some of these oils are extracted and condensed by a very simple process, while some require a complicated procedure for proper extraction. The process to make some of these oils can be just a little too complex to be used at home.

Many of the more popular essential oils can be purchased, off the shelf, in most drugstores, herbal and health stores, as well as on the web and at very reasonable prices.

Below this temperature the active components are released intact. On the other hand, if the producer uses a higher temperature than 180F a significant portion of the essence of the plant components will be broken down and released into the air. When this is the case, these oils will not have as strong an affect when used to treat health issues.

Essential Oil and Notes

Essential Oils aromas are used when categorizing them as being in different classifications or "Notes".

Top Note Oils have a pleasing light and fruity or flowery aroma.

Base Note Oils on the other hand, have very spicy and earthy or even pungent aromas which are typically not a pleasing as a Top Note Oil.

172

Middle Note Oils are a grouping of oils that characterized as having aromas that are between Top and Base Note Oils.

Blending Essential Oils – Using Notes

To properly blend different Essential Oils and still have an aroma where no one oil overpowers the others in the mixture, it is recommended that the Oils be blended by combining Notes in the following manner;

When you are blending oils try to use a combination of: 3-part Top Note Oil, 2-parts Middle Note Oil and 1-part Base Note Oil together and you will typically get a balanced combination of aromas.

Tips for using Essential Oils

Always shake your essential oils thoroughly before using them as many have ingredients that will separate and settle over time.

Store your oils in Amber colored bottles, well sealed and away from sunlight. This is because many oils are photosensitive and will degrade faster if exposed to sunlight. Using amber or other colored bottles will slow down their degradation.

As with many conventional medicines, a person's overexposure to a specific Essential Oil for a long period of time can reduce its effectiveness.

You will often find that you can purchase your essential oils online to get the best price, if you are not making them yourself.

See the section in Book-III of The Retro-Survivalist called; HERBs, FRUITs, PLANTs and their BENEFITS for detailed descriptions of the plants many of the more popular Essential Oils are made from.

Essential Oil Warnings

As the personal use of Essential Oils has become more popular, there have a growing number of manufacturers of products that they call Essential Oils. Many are truly that but; some are weak reflections of the real thing.

Before purchasing these products read the label and the listing of the actual ingredients in the bottle. Often you will see long chemical names where they have substituted or added other chemicals that are not the true and pure essential oil that you may be expecting.

True Essential Oils are typically very concentrated and they should be used with caution both externally and especially internally, and even then, only as directed.

Topical Use – Because the skin of some people can be extremely sensitive to some chemicals, topical application of essential oils should be done only when diluted.

Dilute the oil as directed, before application. Many oils listed as safe are often diluted with other vegetable oils such as Almond Oil or Avocado Oil.

SKIN REACTIONS: If you are unsure about a person's skin reaction to specific Essential Oils, apply a small amount to the skin and wait for a reaction such as redness, itching or a rash to occur.

Typically, you would never use more than six drops of an Essential Oil on the skin. And of course, you should never use an essential oil on mucous membranes, in the ear, and especially not on or near the eyes.

Because so many essential oils are photosensitive, you should never apply these to the skin and then go out into the sun.

If a negative reaction does occur, wash the oil away with a vegetable oil such as Almond Oil, Avocado Oil, Sunflower Oil, etc. to dilute the negative reaction to the essential oil.

Internal Consumption – Essential Oils are typically not recommended for internal consumption. The exceptions are when they are labeled as being diluted and prepared for use as a Dietary Supplement, or when they are specifically labeled as being safe for use in the treatment of certain health problems.

When this is the case, follow the instructions for use precisely.

Popular ESSENTIAL OILS

The following list includes some of the more popular Essential Oils and information on how they are to be used.

Basil Oil

This oil is a Top Note and has a fresh sweet smelling yet spicy aroma. Basil Oil is **photosensitive** so you should not use it in mixtures that will be applied to the skin that might be exposed to the Sun.

It mixes well with Bergamot and Clary Sage Oils and is used in aromatherapy to treat; **Anxiety, Depression** and **Fatigue** while boosting mental clarity.

This Oil should be properly diluted if applied topically. If taken internally, it must be diluted properly and if it is commercially produced it must labeled as a dietary supplement.

Basil is often used to provide relief with such problems as **fluid retention, head colds, kidney conditions, stomach spasms** and **gas**. Women use Basil to **improve blood circulation after childbirth.**

Bergamot Oil

Bergamot Oil is an essential oil and has a light, refreshing aroma of Oranges and flowers.

It is used as an **antibiotic**, an **analgesic**, a **stimulant** and an **anti-depressant.**

Often it is used as an Insect Repellant as well as to treat such health problems as; Acne, Eczema and Insect bites. In Aromatherapy it has a good mood balancing scent. It mixes well with Citrus, Lavender, Rose and Sage Oils

Canola Oil

There is no Canola tree or plant. It is actually Rapeseed Oil but when the FDA banned the use of Rapeseed Oil, the name was changed by the Canadian production company for marketing purposes. See Rapeseed Oil.

Castor Oil

Castor Oil is extracted from the beans (or seeds) of the Castor plant; which grows in tropical regions worldwide. **The Castor seed contains Ricin (a toxin)** that is inactivated during the extraction process of the oil.

The oil can be used as a **stimulant, laxative** and typically **results in digestive purging within 4-6 hours.**

It has been successfully used to **dissolve cysts, some types of tumors, skin tags, warts** and even **moles.**

WARNING: Castor Oil is often used as a **skin moisturizer,** especially on dry and mature skin but it **can cause skin reactions, diarrhea and cramps** for some people.

Donald W Bobbitt

Cedar Wood Oil

Cedar Wood Oil is a Low Note and has a strong woodsy scent.

The Oil is made from the wood and roots and often the foliage of conifer trees, typically Pine and Cypress trees.

Cedar Wood Essential Oil is used as an **astringent, antiseptic, anti-inflammatory, anti-spasmodic, diuretic, expectorant, sedative**, and to treat such problems as **eczema** and **arthritic pain**

It can be used topically undiluted and for internal use, but it must be diluted and labeled as such and safe for consumption when used internally.

WARNING: The use of Cedar Wood Oil should be avoided during pregnancy and used only in low doses. It **can cause nausea, vomiting and thirst** and even **damage to the digestive system** if taken in large doses.

The Oil is a **strong pesticide** and was **used in embalming** for thousands of years because of this. Cedar Wood Oil is a good insect repellant. It has **anti-fungal** and **anti-bacterial** properties making it a very **good cleaning agent**.

Chamomile Oil

Chamomile Oil is extracted form the flowers of the Chamomile plant. This essential oil has an herb-like, sweet scent and it is often used in shampoos.

Chamomile Oil has **antiseptic, anti-spasmodic, analgesic, anti-bacterial, anti-neuralgic** and **antibiotic** properties. It is used in an herbal infusion to treat **insomnia**. It is also used to treat; **Acne, Insect Bites, Skin Rash, Sunburn** and other **Sensitive skin problems**.

It can be used topically undiluted and for internal use, it must be labeled as being safe for consumption.

WARNING: Pregnant women should not use Chamomile Oil, as it can cause uterine contractions and could cause a miscarriage.

Cilantro Oil

Cilantro, itself has a fresh flavor favored in cooking recipes. Cilantro Oil comes from the leaves of the Coriander plant. It must be diluted whether it is used topically or internally.

Cilantro Oil has **antioxidant** properties, enhances the **digestive process**, and is a **strong stimulant**.

Toxic Metal purging: Taking 1-2 drops of Cilantro Oil (in a capsule) 4 times a day for up to 4-weeks internally will help remove toxic metals, such as Mercury, Aluminum, Tin, and Lead, from the brain, spinal cord and fatty tissues of body. Once the metal is mobilized it is excreted via the stool and urine.

Cinnamon Bark Oil

Cinnamon Oil is an aromatic essential oil with a spicy scent. It has **anti-microbial** properties and is a **natural stimulant**.

This oil is used to **prevent the spread of germs** and to **fight mental fatigue** as well as **depression**.

WARNING: It blends well with Citrus oils but **can be a skin irritant** if used in sprays and applied too thickly to the skin. It should only be used on or by, Adults and then only when it is properly diluted.

Clary Sage Oil

Clary Sage Oil is extracted from the Clary Sage plant that is native to European countries. It is a Base Note and has an earthy, pungent odor. It is used as a muscatel flavoring in wines and liqueurs.

Like its scent, this oil is strong and should be used in small amounts.

It is an **antioxidant** and has **antiseptic** properties. It is often used as an **anti-depressant** as well as to **stimulate Hormone production** in the body.

Clove Oil

Clove Oil is extracted from the leaves of the Clove plant.

It is a good **analgesic** and **antiseptic** used for centuries by dentists. It contains eugenol that works well to sooth **toothaches**. It is also a good **anti-bacterial** and **anti-microbial**.

Coconut Oil

Coconut Oil is made from the white meat inside the Coconut shell

CAUTION: Large doses can cause vomiting, nausea, digestive tract pain, sore throats, rapid heartbeat and dizziness.

and is actually considered Base Oil. With its great flavor and aroma it is used widely in cooking and cosmetic applications

---

CAUTION: Use only organic, Virgin or Cold-processed versions of Coconut Oil to treat health issues.

Coconut Oil will melt at 76F and works well in both liquid and paste forms. It contains saturated fats, but the fat is a **Lactic Acid based fat**. The fatty acids make your hair feel silky and soft as well as reducing frizz.

Be aware that many refined Coconut Oils have been bleached and heated and will have lost most of its medicinal properties, so these are best used for cooking and not Health issues.

Coconut Oil has a number of health benefits, including; **helping with weight loss**. It can also **help the body fight streptococcus bacteria**.

Coconut Oil has strong natural **anti-bacterial, anti-fungal, anti-microbial**, and **anti-viral** properties and is also a great skin moisturizer.

Coconut Oil can be used as a teeth whitener when used in the Ayurvedic technique called Oil pulling, which involved rinsing your mouth for 10-20 minutes with a teaspoon of coconut oil before brushing your teeth.

Cypress Oil

Cypress Oil is extracted from the leaves and cones of the Cypress tree. It has a strong woodsy scent. It is a good insect repellant and helps in treating oily skin.

Cypress Oil can be used undiluted topically but should not be used al all internally.

It is a very **strong astringent** and is used often to treat such health issues as **hemorrhoids** (in a 1 to 2% diluted wash), **varicose veins** (a small dosage applied very lightly, no rubbing), **arthritic pain, colds** and **influenza, diarrhea, menstrual problems**, and **muscle pains**.

> **CAUTION**: this oil can irritate the skin if used in high doses, also do not use this oil if you are pregnant.

It also has medicinal applications due to these natural properties, as it is an **anti-bacterial, antibiotic, antiseptic, disinfectant,** and a **sedative**.

Eugenol

Eugenol is an essential oil blend most often made by combining the essential oils of Bay leaves with Clove Oil, Basil Oil, Nutmeg Oil and/or Cinnamon Oil to name the ones with the higher concentrations.

Eugenol is rich in **antioxidants** and has **strong antiseptic and anesthetic properties**. It is used most often in dentistry to numb the pain of **toothaches**.

It is also used as an aid in the treatment of **digestive problems**, to help **treat influenza**, to **relieve heartburn**, and to **cover up bad breath**.

> **Warning**: Use Eugenol only as directed as an overdose can cause damage to the Liver.

Echinacea

Echinacea, also called **American Coneflower**, is a flowering plant in the Daisy family. It thrives in dry prairies and open woodlands. It is also a popular herb native to North America.

Echinacea has **antibiotic** properties that make it quite useful when applied to the skin to **treat burns, boils, eczema, psoriasis, bee stings and sunburns**.

Echinacea tincture is purported to be **effective aiding in the cure of Chicken Pox** and **Shingles**. It acts as a **stimulant** for the **body's immune system** and is widely used for its antibiotic properties.

Because Echinacea stimulates the body's immune system it is often used to **fight urinary tract infections, vaginal yeast infections and such other infections as; tonsillitis, syphilis, malaria, typhoid, migraine headaches, acid indigestion, tooth pain** from infection and other pains.

Eucalyptus Oil

Eucalyptus Oil is made from the leaves of the Eucalyptus tree, which was originally found in Australia.

This Oil has **anti-bacterial** and **anti-viral** properties and is often used in the treatment of **common colds, Influenza,** and **nasal congestion** (through steam inhalation) as well as for treating **muscle pains** and **joint pain** (mixed into bath waters) and for **nasal congestion.**

This Oil is available in several types including **Peppermint Eucalyptus Oil** that has a Mint-like scent and **Bay Gum Eucalyptus Oil** that has a pungent woodsy scent. Bay Gum Eucalyptus Oil is often used to treat **muscle pains.**

Evening Primrose Oil

The essential oil of the Evening Primrose, which is made from the bark and the leaves of the plant by the same name, is used in a number of medicinal applications.

It is purported to **help fight certain Cancers** and to treat such ailments as; **acne, arthritic pain, brittle nails, hyperactivity, premenstrual tension** and even **multiple sclerosis** and **liver damage.**

The roots can be made into a poultice and applied to **bruises** and by making a tea from the roots; it is used to **treat stomach pain** and **bowel pain.**

FLAX SEED Oil

Flax Seed Oil is also known as Mucilage. Mucilage is produced by boiling Golden Flax seeds in a mixture with water and then extracting the liquid from the mixture.

Flax Seed Oil is a useful treatment for such ailments as Sinus problems, **Lung congestion, coughs,** and even for easing **joint pains.**

Frankincense Oil

Frankincense Oil is a Middle Note and has a strong aromatic scent. It has been made from the Herb by the same name for thousands of years.

It is used as an **anti-inflammatory.**

It mixes well with Basil, Bergamot, Cinnamon, Lavender, Orange and Sandalwood, to name a few other Oils.

Geranium Oil

Although there are over 700 varieties of the plant itself, the stems and bark of less than ten are used to extract this Essential Oil. Its major use is in aromatherapy to stimulate the adrenal system, balance the hormonal system and balance the mind and emotions.

Geranium Oil has the a number of health applications including being an; **astringent**, being a **styptic** which causes bleeding to stop in wounds, aids in the healing of **wounds** and the **formation of scars,** improves **aging skin**, and as a **vermifuge** in that it aids in the body destroying and expelling **parasitic worms**.

It is also used to treat; **acne, burns, cuts, dermatitis, eczema, hemorrhoids, lice, ringworm, ulcers, edema, poor circulation, sore throat, tonsillitis, PMS, menopause** problems as well as **stress** and **neuralgia.**

Geranium Oil can be used undiluted topically, is generally safe for kids, and can be used internally if properly diluted.

Ginger Oil

Ginger Root Oil is made from the Ginger root itself and its strength depends on the quality of the Ginger Root as well as the distillation process used. It is an essential oil with a Middle Note that has a fresh and spicy scent often used in Colognes.

Ginger Root Oil has a number of useful properties including being an **analgesic, anti-inflammatory, antiseptic** and having **carminative properties** (it causes the expulsion of gas from the digestive tract).

It is used to aid in the treatment of such health issues as; **inflammation, digestive problems, indigestion, irregular and painful menstrual problems, heart problems, respiratory problems and nausea.**

It can also be used to help treat **food poisoning, respiratory problems such as colds, flu, asthma, and bronchitis** and is **very good at removing mucous from the lungs and throat.**

It is used in some parts of the world for treating other problems such as **dissolving kidney stones, treating some Cancers, managing stress** and even **curing malaria attacks.**

Donald W Bobbitt

Ginger Oil can be used topically or internally if properly diluted. Ginger Tea works well for relieving stomach problems.

CAUTION: Ginger Oil can be a skin irritant to some people.

Grapefruit Oil

Grapefruit Oil is a Top Note essential oil with a refreshing, yet short-lived, scent. The oil is a natural antiseptic, disinfectant, diuretic and stimulant.

It is often used to treat such situations as **anorexia, digestive problems, dry throat, Liver disorders, migraine headaches and PMS** as well as **helping heal acne, and other skin problems.**

Grapefruit Oil is **photosensitive** so you should not use it in mixtures that will be applied to the skin that might be exposed to the Sun. This oil should be properly diluted if applies topically. If taken internally, it normally doesn't have to be diluted.

Hyssop Oil

Hyssop leaves have a bitter, minty flavor and is used most often in Colognes as well as in the liquors Chartreuse and Absinthe.

It has anti-inflammatory properties and is used, in conjunction with other herbs to make herbal remedies for **lung congestion and other health conditions**. Its use can help **strengthen the immune system**.

Hyssop Oil can be used topically or internally if properly diluted.

Jasmine Oil

Jasmine Oil is an Absolute Oil and not actually an Essential Oil because the flowers are too delicate to survive the distillation process used to make most essential oils.

Jasmine Oil is made by laying the flowers out on a clean cotton cloth and then soaked in Olive oil for several days. Then the oil is extracted (usually pressed and filtered) giving the true essence called Jasmine Oil.

Jasmine Oil is used as an **antiseptic, anti-depressant, a sedative, and an expectorant** and it is a **good disinfectant.** For women, It can ease **menstrual pains**. It also eases the pains of **rheumatism**.

Jasmine oil can be used undiluted topically and can be used internally if labeled as a dietary supplement.

Lavender Oil

Lavender Oil is a very popular essential oil extracted from the flowers of the plant using a steam distillation process.. It is a Top note and has a distinctly sweet floral scent.

The oil blends well with a number of other essential oils such as Cedar Wood, Citrus, Pine, Sage and Rosemary.

In **aromatherapy** it blends well with Rosemary and is used to keep one **feeling alert and calm.** It also **soothes headaches**.

Lavender Oil can help **treat burns** on areas of the skin, and to **control bleeding** from cuts. One drop of Lavender Oil on the tongue can help reduce **motion sickness**.

One drop on a **cold sore** will speed up the healing process. It is useful to ease pain and relieve nervous tension and it helps improve blood circulation and to help treat respiratory problems.

Lavender Oil can be used undiluted topically and can be used internally if labeled as a dietary supplement. It is also considered to be generally safe for children.

It also makes a good **insect repellant**.

Lemon Oil

Lemon Oil is an Essential Oil that has a fresh fruity fragrance. It is used to sooth **respiratory problems** such as **Bronchitis, Colds and Sore Throats**.

It blends well with other Citrus Oils Lavender, Rose and Sandalwood Oils.

Lemon Oil is **photosensitive** so you should not use it topically if the area of the skin might be exposed to the Sun.

This Oil should be properly diluted if applies topically. If taken internally, it must be diluted properly and if it is commercially produced it must labeled as a dietary supplement.

Lemongrass Oil

Lemongrass Oil is an essential oil with a citrus-like, yet herbal scent.

It blends well with Lavender and should be used sparingly to avoid an overpowering odor. Used in aromatherapy it is relaxing and uplifting.

It also blends well with Bergamot, Patchouli and Rosemary Oils.

Lemongrass Oil is steam extracted and has **antioxidant, anti-fungal** and **anti-bacterial** properties.

Lemongrass Oil is used for a number of health issues including; **reducing high fevers and alleviating pains such as; digestive tract spasms, muscle spasms,** and **stomach problems.** It is reputed to; **improve blood circulation, contribute to pancreatic health, treat digestive issues** and is said to **contribute to killing Cancer cells.**

Lemongrass Oil must be diluted whether it is used topically or internally, and is only for use by adults.

It is an excellent **insect repellant** while on the other hand; it is often used to lure hiving Honey Bees.

Lemon Verbena Oil

This oil is extracted from the fresh leaves of the plant via steam distillation. It is an Essential Oil and a Top note with a fresh fruity scent. It is often used to add a Lemon flavor to Fish and other dishes.

This oil has **antioxidant** properties as well as being used as; an **antiseptic, digestive aid, an emollient, a sedative** and is often used to treat such problems as **Anxiety** and **Insomnia.**

Lime Oil

Lime Oil is an essential oil and a Top note with a pleasing fruity and sweet scent. The oil is extracted by squeezing it from the rinds of Limes.

It blends well with Basil in most applications.

Lime Oil is used as; an **antiseptic, anti-bacterial,** and **anti-viral.** The Oil is often used to treat such problems as **Acne, Colds, Fevers, Liver detoxification, Sore Throats, Insect Bites and Oily Skin.**

To purify drinking water, add a drop of the oil to a glass of water.

Mint Oil

Mint Oil is an essential oil with a strong Minty fragrance. It is often used in toothpastes and mouth washes to **cleanse the mouth by killing germs** and providing **fresh breath.**

RECIPE: How to make Mint Oil;
1- Pick fresh Mint leaves,

2- Pack the leaves into a sealable jar,

3- Cover the leaves with Vodka,

4- Seal the jar and allow to sit in a warm area for at least two weeks,

5- Strain the liquid and freeze the liquid.

6- After freezing, remove the upper portion, which will be the Vodka and pour the lower part (the Mint Oil itself) into an amber bottle.

7- Seal the bottle and use it when needed. It will keep for 6-12 months.

Commercial Mint Oil (the more pure versions) must be diluted whether it is used topically or internally, and is only for use by adults.

MUCILAGE

Mucilage is another name for Flax Seed Oil. Mucilage is a natural oil useful for treating such problems as **Lung Congestion, Coughs, Eczema, and Sinus problems**. It is also used to help **ease joint pain**.

RECIPE: How to make Mucilage,

a.   Bring 2-cups of water to a boil

b.   Add 2-tbs. of whole Flax Seeds to the water.

c.   Reduce the temperature as low as possible and bring the mixture to a boil again.

d.   Keep the mixture at a low boil for 7-8 minutes or until the water begins to thicken.

e.   Remove from the heat and allow the mixture to cool. It should resemble a thick liquid with white streaks in it that resemble egg whites.

f.   Pour the liquid into an amber colored glass jar, seal the jar and store in the fridge for up to 10-days. Like most homemade oils Mucilage will go bad (turn Rancid) within 8-10-days.

The Oil has a slimy taste and many people add it to other flavorful drinks, baked goods and even main dishes to mask its taste.

There is one variety of Flax Seed Oil that is known as Linseed Oil and it is not to be taken internally as it is poisonous. Another variety of Flax Seed Oil is not good for your lungs and the user should read the different labels carefully to make sure that they are using the appropriate oil.

It is recommended that new users of Mucilage try only 1-tsp as a first dose to make sure that their stomachs can handle the effects of the oil. If all is well the next day, they can then increase the dosage.

Donald W Bobbitt

MULLEIN Oil

Mullein Oil is made from the Great Mullein plant that is found throughout Europe, Asia and North America.

It is a good **astringent, anti-inflammatory, emollient** and **demulcent** and has some **slightly sedative** and even **narcotic properties**.

MULLEIN OIL, Make your own

RECIPE-1; How to make Mullein Oil,

It will take about one-half cup (4 ounces) of fresh Mullein flowers (yellow in color) to make almost one-half cup (4 ounces) of Mullein Oil.

1- Place the flowers in a jar and cover them with EVOO (Extra Virgin Olive Oil),
2- Cover the jar with a lid and seal well.
3- Then set the jar on a sunny window for a month (28-30 days, usually).
4- Strain the contents of the jar into another clean jar using a cloth or even a paper coffee filter.
5- After the liquid sits for an hour or so, you will notice some moisture drops settled at the bottom of the jar.
6- Slowly drain the liquid into a third jar leaving the bottom layer of liquid containing the moisture drops behind.
7- Any remnant of water will make the moisture spoil.
8- Finally, seal the jar of Mullin Oil well until needed.
9- Some of the Oil can be placed in a clean dry eyedropper bottle for ease of use.

RECIPE-2: A simple Mullein Oil infusion can be made by boiling 1- oz. of dried leaves in 1- pint of milk for 10-minutes.

RECIPE-3: The dried leaves can be smoked in a regular tobacco pipe to relieve the hacking cough of Consumption.

RECIPE-4: Steep the flowers of the plant in Olive Oil for at least 3- weeks to make a strong bactericide.

MYRRH Oil

Myrrh Oil is an Essential Oil and is a Low note with a spicy scent. It blends well with Frankincense, Lavender, Mints and Sandalwood oils.

Myrrh is often used as an **astringent** and **anti-fungal**.

Myrrh Oil can be used undiluted topically and can be used internally if labeled as a dietary supplement. It is also considered to be generally safe for children.

NUTMEG Oil

Nutmeg Oil is made via a steam distillation process from Nutmeg powder or dried seeds.

This oil is used primarily for **treating nervous system and digestive system problems**. The Oil can be used similar to Clove oil to **ease toothaches**.

Add 3-4 drops to 1-tsp. of honey to treat nausea, gastroenteritis, indigestion as well as chronic diarrhea.

It can be used in a massage oil to treat muscle pains, arthritic pain, gout, and rheumatism.

NOTE: Nutmeg Oil must be diluted whether it is used topically or internally.

OLIVE Oil

Olive Oil is actually considered a Base Oil and is made by pressing the oil from whole Olives. It is used widely in cooking applications around the world for its flavor.

Olive Oil is high **in antioxidants** and is used in certain health applications, such as; **healing ear infections, lowering cholesterol levels, reducing the risk of certain cancers and treating some skin problems.**

It is a good **skin moisturizer** and **helps with dry hair**. Regular consumption of Olive oil also helps **control blood sugar levels**.

Long-term consumption of Extra Virgin Olive Oil is purported to be one reason for **reduced instances of Heart problems** in some countries where the population eats a "Mediterranean Diet".

USDA Grades for Olive Oil

Olive Oil is popular around the world and most of the honest manufacturers and distributors follow a standard grading and labeling system for their products.

But, there are some distributors who try to pass lower grades of Olive Oil for the better and more expensive ones. See **Table B2-2** for a list of the **Major Grades of Olive Oils**.

Donald W Bobbitt

OLIVE LEAF Extract

The oils extracted from Olive leaves has strong **anti-inflammatory** and **antibiotic** properties and they also have **antioxidant** levels that are over two times that of Green Tea and four times that of Vitamin C from fruits.

Olive Leaf Extract has proven to be useful in treating such health problems as *High Blood Pressure*, as well as **some Cancers** and **other tumors**.

ORANGE Oil

Orange Oil is an essential oil with a sweet fragrance like the Orange fruit itself.

The oil is a natural **antiseptic** and **anti-bacterial**. It is used in **aromatherapy** as an **anti-depressant**. It blends well with; other Citrus oils, Lavender, Patchouli, Rosemary and Sage Oils.

Orange Oil is **photosensitive** so you should not use it topically if the area of the skin might be exposed to the Sun.

This Oil should be properly diluted if applies topically. If taken internally, it must be diluted properly. It is also considered to be generally safe for children.

OREGANO Oil

Oregano Oil is extracted from the plant of the herb Oregano through steam distillation. It has **anti-fungal, anti-inflammatory, anti-microbial, anti-viral**, and **anti-parasitic** properties.

It has been used, in diluted form, to treat such health problems as; **upper Gastro-intestinal problems, colds, influenza, candida, skin problems, nail fungus, joint pain**, and **dandruff**

WARNING: Oregano Oil must be diluted whether it is used topically or internally, and is only for use by adults.

PATCHOULI Oil

Patchouli Oil is an expensive essential oil and a Low Note that has a rich lasting scent.

Patchouli Oil is used to treat; **acne, athlete's foot, dermatitis, eczema** and other **skin problems**.

It is also used as an **aphrodisiac** and is a good **insect repellant**.

Patchouli Oil can be used topically and internally in undiluted form and is generally considered safe for children.

PEPPERMINT Oil

Peppermint is actually a hybrid cross between **Spearmint** and **Watermint**. Peppermint Oil is an essential oil and is a Top Note with a very refreshing minty aroma and has also been used in culinary dishes for hundreds of years.

It has been used for centuries to treat such problems as **abdominal pains, indigestion, irritable bowel, nausea**, and **vomiting**. It is used in **aromatherapy** and its pleasing aroma is purported to enhance the memory and mental alertness.

It is an **anti-spasmodic** and **anti-bacterial**, and its high level of the chemical *pulegone* make it a good pesticide. It is used to ease heartburn and inflammation in the mouth and throat. It can help ease toothaches and headaches.

WARNING: The oil **can be an irritant to the stomach** if not used in low doses, and should not be used on children.

NOTE: Peppermint Oil also repels Mosquitos.

PINE Oil

Pine Oil is an essential oil that has a fresh invigorating Pine scent. It is made by steam distilling the needles, cones and even twigs of several different pine trees.

It is a natural **antiseptic, anti-microbial, anti-bacterial** and **anti-viral** treatment tool. In **aromatherapy** it is used to **relieve stress**, and **fight fatigue**.

It blends well with; bergamot, lavender, lemon, rosemary and tea tree oils, to name a few.

CAUTION: Pine Oil can cause breathing problems for some people, and can irritate the skin and mucous membranes.

It used in household cleansers for its aroma.

RAPESEED OIL

Oilcan RAPESEED Oil is also known as **Rape, Rapa, Rapeseed, Oilseed** and **Canola Oil**.

The original Rapeseed Oil was such a strong toxin when used in large doses that the FDA banned it for human consumption in 1956.

In 1970 Canadian growers developed a new form of Rapeseed oil that was lower in erucic oil and gave it a new name, Canola, which is short for Canadian Oil Low Acid.

Canola Oil is **low in saturated fats** and **high in monounsaturated fatty acids**.

WARNING: Canola Oil has a weak flavor and it contains high levels of the chemical, **erucic acid**, which has been **found to be damaging to heart muscles**. Canola Oil is regulated by the FDA and must contain less than 2% erucic oil in the USA while the EU allows up to 5%.

The oil is also a great **pesticide**.

ROSEMARY Oil

Rosemary Oil is an essential oil and is a Middle note with a refreshing aroma. The oil is made from fresh Rosemary leaves.

It is high in antioxidants, has disinfectant properties and makes a great mouthwash and it has antiseptic properties and is often used in the treatment of; **acne, dandruff, indigestion, respiratory problems, oily hair** and is even said to promote hair growth.

It is used to **relieve pains** such as **headaches, rheumatism** and **arthritic pain.** It is a decent **diuretic** and It is even used to reduce the **inflammation** of the **recurring herpes virus**.

In **aromatherapy** it is used to **fight depression, exhaustion, headaches, and stress.**

It blends well with basil, lavender, lemongrass and pine oils. Rosemary Oil must be diluted whether it is used topically or internally, and is only for use by adults.

SANDALWOOD Oil

Sandalwood Oil is an essential oil and is a Low Note and a long-lasting woodsy aroma. It has been used for thousands of years for its unique scent.

The oil is an aromatic used in **aromatherapy**. Sandalwood oil is often used in cosmetics, soaps and numerous skin care products. It is often used medicinally for its **expectorant, anti-inflammatory, antiseptic, diuretic** and **sedative** properties.

The full strength oil is a **good expectorant** and also works well to **treat bronchitis** and this can be done several ways.

RECIPE: Place 5-6 drops onto a sugar cube or over a teaspoon of sugar or even over a teaspoon of honey. Then place the mixture into your mouth and allow it to slowly slide down your throat. Repeat this twice daily.

Sandalwood Oil can be used undiluted topically and can be used internally if labeled as a dietary supplement. It is also considered to be generally safe for children.

SESAME Seed Oil

Sesame Oil is extracted from dried, ripened Sesame seeds. The seeds themselves are high in such nutrients as; Vitamins E, B1, calcium, magnesium, iron, Phosphorous, molybdenum, selenium and copper and it's popular in many culinary dishes, especially in Asia.

The oil has a number of reputed health applications, such as being an **anti-bacterial, anti-inflammatory** and an **anti-fungal**.

It is known for being; **a skin massage oil**, working well to **reduce plaque and whiten teeth** via the "oil Pulling" technique, **lowering blood pressure** and **cholesterol, reducing type-2 diabetes sugar levels** aids in **reducing the effects of radiation from X-Rays, aids in the prevention of some cancers**.

SPEARMINT Oil

This essential oil that has a warm Minty aroma. The oil is extracted by using a distillation process with the flowers of the plant.

It has been used for centuries as an **antiseptic** and **stimulant** and also is reputed to have **astringent** and **anti-spasmodic** properties. It also is used to **reduce menstrual pains** and to **reduce the associated nausea, fatigue** and **abdominal pain.**

It blends well with basil, jasmine and rosemary oils. Spearmint Oil must be diluted whether it is used topically or internally, and is only for use by adults.

SWEET ORANGE Oil

Sweet Orange Oil is an essential oil and is a Top note with a light Citrusy aroma that dissipates quickly. It is used as a flavoring in beverages and some culinary recipes.

The oil is used for its; **anti-inflammatory** and **antiseptic** properties and it even aids in **combating the growth of cancer tumors.**

It blends well with a number of other oils such as Clove Oil.

TANGERINE Oil

Tangerine Oil is extracted from the peel of the Tangerine fruit.

It is often used for its health benefits and properties such as being **anti-spasmodic,** a **sedative, aiding in cell regeneration** and in **removing toxins** from the blood. It is used to treat **diarrhea, rashes, dry skin**, and eases **constipation**.

The oil is **photosensitive** so you should not use it topically if the area of the skin might be exposed to the Sun.

This oil should be properly diluted if applies topically. If taken internally, it must be diluted properly.

TEA TREE Oil

Tea Tree Oil is an essential oil with a fresh but medicinal aroma. It's made from the leaves, twigs and the bark of the tree is a valuable medicinal tool.

This Oil is a great **antiseptic, anti-bacterial, anti-microbial** and **anti-fungal** medical tool that is a stimulant to the immune system.

It is used to treat; **acne, athlete's foot, burns, chronic fatigue syndrome, cold sores, cystitis, glandular fever, insect bitess, nits, thrush, vaginal infections, cerrucae** and **warts**.

In **aromatherapy** it's used to **ease respiratory problems** and for **clearing the head**. It blends well with lavender, lemon, mint and rosemary oils.

THYME Oil

Thyme is a common Herb often used as a spice or condiment. The Oil is extracted using a steam distillation process on the fresh flowers and leaves of the plant.

It has some very useful health benefits due to the following properties. It is a good **antiseptic, anti-rheumatic, anti-spasmodic, diuretic, stimulant,** and **expectorant**.

It is good for treating, Coughs, colds, convulsions, cramps and aches due to spasms, as well as epileptic attacks. Being a **diuretic**, it removes toxins from the body and relieves arthritis, rheumatism and even gout pain.

Thyme contains Camphene, and Carophyllene which make it a good antiseptic for wounds and cuts. As an **anti-spasmodic** it is useful to calm the heart and relaxes arteries and veins thus lowering blood pressure.

For women it gives relief by helping open up obstructed menses reducing pain from abdominal spasms, fatigue and nausea during menstruation.

YLANG YLANG Oil

Ylang Ylang Oil is made from the flower by the same name.

It has a number of medicinal properties including being an; anti-depressant, antiseptic, anti-seborrhic, aphrodisiac, as well as being a good sedative.

 It can be used undiluted topically and can be used internally if labeled as a dietary supplement. It's also considered to be safe for topical use with children.

Don't go OFF THE GRID, just head to the edge.

Everything that you have read, so far, in this book, was included to help you become a more knowledgeable and self-sufficient person or family.

You have read how to, at least know what is in those prepared and canned foods and medicines that are thrust at you in the supermarkets and pharmacies that you frequent.

You have been given information on ways to take control not only of what you buy and consume, but also some alternative ways to grow and raise some of your own foods, if you so desire.

And, you have been given a number of common and effective ways to treat a number of the illnesses and health problems that people incur most often. These treatments use natural ingredients that have been used by people around the world for centuries.

And, if you find that need them, there are instruction for making some of these treatments, poultices, tinctures and other medicines yourself.

So, if you want to actually drop off of the Grid, what is in this book will not get you there, but it will give you information on a few of the easier and simpler things that one of those serious Off-the-Grid people will need or already know.

That is why I coined the term RETRO-SURVIVALIST. These are truly "retro" tools, ideas, and methods for you to use and simplify things for yourself and make your life a healthier one.

To go "Off Grid" requires one to make some major and costly commitments to get there. These commitments include:

STUDY How to be SELF SUFFICIENT

Essentially, you need to understand the level of commitment needed to be not just a farmer but also one who raises and grows ALL of their own foods. You see, to be Off the Grid means that in good and bad weather, when you are off of the grid. Regardless of outside conditions, you are an isolated family or person who lives and farms without many of the technological tools or toys available today.

You will be living a very simple lifestyle and you will inherently be isolated from much of society.

You need Special SKILLS

A self-sufficient person living off of the grid has to be a jack-of-all-trades. He must:

1. Be an **Architect** and know how to make furniture, build a home, barn and other buildings,
2. Be a **Horticulturalist** in order to grow and protect their crops from pests.
3. Be a **Veterinarian** in order to care for and raise healthy Cattle, Pigs, Chickens, etc.
4. Be an **Electrical Engineer** in order to efficiently install and repair Solar Power Systems, Water Pumps, Light systems, etc.
5. Be a **Hydraulics Engineer** in order to design and manage the flow of Land-water, Lake Water, and Creek Water to keep their crops and animals watered properly.
6. Be a **Financial Manager** who knows how to manage their crops for maximum output in order to not only survive, but to have enough extra to trade with others for the consumable essentials you will need to keep their farm viable each year.

Add to these skills the serious Survivalist must have a broad knowledge of other necessary professions like; Butcher, Meat Packager, Food Handler and Packer, Pest Control Manager, Chemical Engineer, Tool Maker, Tractor and Truck Mechanic, Waste Management Specialist, Roofer, Insulator, Plumber, Physical Therapist, Physician, Dentist, and on and on.

Reasons to just head to the EDGE of the GRID

I recommend that you do the things that you can do that will make your life and your family happier. Do the things that you can do, over time that improves the quality of your life.

As you work your way towards the Edge of the Grid and take over many of the facets of your life and health, you will, in all probability enjoy the following benefits;

WORK FEWER hours on your job in order to sustain a quality lifestyle.

REDUCE STRESS that you and your family suffer from by competing so hard to get by in a convoluted and unforgiving society.

SET NEW STANDARDS in your life that better define what you really need and want.

Donald W Bobbitt

LIVE A HEALTHIER LIFE by understanding what you are putting into your body and what the effects are on your body.

MANAGE YOUR HEALTH by understanding natural treatments for common health problems that you can utilize and not be exposed to potentially dangerous chemicals.

BE HAPPY – Yes, if you are in control of your life and health, are spending your food and medicine dollars more intelligently, and then you will definitely be happier.

Your foods will be safer and under your control and not products that of corporations who push GMOs at us.

Your job will be something that allows you to make enough money to raise a healthier family at a lower cost and not to keep up with the wealthy.

You'll eat less often at fast-food restaurants and more often at home. You and your family will be able to cook healthier meals; real meals made of real and natural ingredientss whenever possible.

You will be more aware of your use of Fossil Fuels and you will be doing your part by using them intelligently and sparingly as you go through life.

You will probably own one or more guns along with ammunition for them. These guns will be designed for hunting, but if the time comes when you need to defend your land and your family, they would also work well for self-defense.

You will continue to own and use computers, but they will be used primarily for research and study, by yourself and your family, to expand your knowledge and not as gaming or social media machines.

You will probably have a backup generator run by gas or solar power. But it will be there to provide the electrical power you need when and if the power grid shuts down, either temporarily of for long periods of time.

Yes, I say be a Retro-Survivalist who knows where the Edge of the Grid happens to be but also knows what works for him and his family and is happy to do the things that work BEST for him.

These things may help you head to a lifestyle that is near the Edge of the Grid, maybe, but definitely not over the Edge.

APPENDIX-A **Dictionary of Words and Phrases used**

Acetic Acid

This is the specific Acid found in Vinegars and is often used for the pickling of foods. Vinegar can contain from 3% to 16% Acetic Acid.

Anti-bacterial

Anti-bacterial is defined as being able to destroy or at least inhibit the growth of bacteria

Antioxidant

Basically, an Antioxidant is a molecule that will inhibit the oxidation of other molecules. The use of antioxidant rich foods is purported to improve heart and other organ health.

Amino ACIDS

Amino Acids are organic compounds that combine in the body to make proteins and they come from foods that we eat. These Amino Acids are used by the body for growth and to break down foods as well as repair body tissues and perform certain bodily functions.

Anthocyanin

Anthocyanins are believed to be active anti-hypertensive compounds, acting as angiotensin-converting enzyme (ACE) inhibitors

Ascorbic Acid

There is natural Ascorbic Acid (or Vitamin-C) and there is industrially created Ascorbic Acid. The industrial version is made from Hydrolyzed Glucose and is called synthetic Vitamin-C. Almost all Ascorbic Acid used in prepared or packaged foods are synthetic.

Aspartame

Aspartame is an artificial sweetener that is used in many packaged foods in place of sugar. The FDA has set the daily safe limit for consumption of Aspartame at 50-mg per 1-kg of body weight.

A typical 12-oz diet soda contains 180-mg of Aspartame. This would convert to a limit of 21 diet sodas for a 165-lb adult. Some side effects of Aspartame, for some people are; headaches, seizures and mood changes.

Astringent

An Astringent is something that causes human tissues to contract. It can help reduce bleeding if applied to a wound.

Calcium Chloride

Calcium Chloride is a salt of Calcium and Chloride. It is used in some prepared foods as a firming agent, specifically in soybean curds to make tofu and canned vegetables. It is also used to reduce the freezing of caramel in candy bars, and to add a salty flavor to foods without raising the actual salt content.

It is estimated that the average American consumes 160-345 mg/day of Calcium Chloride as an additive in prepared foods. The potential side effects of taking Calcium Chloride, are numerous and here are a few; you may be allergic to calcium salts, if you are taking medicines for heart conditions or kidney conditions, if you have low calcium levels, or if you have trouble breathing.

Citric Acid

Citric Acid is a natural acid that is used as a food preservative, a flavoring agent in foods, and to provide an acidic flavor to foods.

Compress

A compress is usually made like a poultice except the liquid part of the mixture is used rather than the herb/plant parts. The liquid is soaked into a soft sterile cloth and thenapplied to the affected area of the body.

Emulsified

An emulsion is a combination of two or more liquids that can normally not be mixed, into an emulsion such as mayonnaise, butter, and vinaigrettes

Expectorant

An expectorant is a class of drugs that promotes hydration. This increased hydration then increases the amount of congestion but the congestion will also be clearer and flow easier. By doing this it lubricates and reduces the irritation of the respiratory tract.

Ferrous Gluconate

Ferrous Gluconate is a compound, black in color that is marketed and used as an Iron supplement and can raise hemoglobin levels relatively quickly in some people.

High levels of Ferrous Gluconate can be toxic so the following daily levels of elemental Iron are recommended; Men – 8-mg, Women – 18-mg, Pregnant Women – 27-mg, and Lactating Women – 9-mg.

Fructose

Fructose is a natural fruit sugar found in many plants such as sugar cane, sugar beets, and corns. When used in foods, the body absorbs it during the digestion process.

Hydrolyzed Vegetable Protein

This chemical is used as a flavor enhancer in gravies, soups, stews and hot dogs among other foods.

Boiling such foods as corn, soy and wheat, among others, in hydrochloric acid and then treating this solution with sodium hydroxide to neutralize it. This breaks the vegetable proteins down into amino acids. One of the amino acids is glutamic acid, in the form of MSG.

Isolate

To isolate a component from a compound such as whey protein, which can be isolated from milk. Whey proteins are digested quickly and are a good source of amino acids. Whey proteins are used after workouts as well as in baby formulas, to aid in growth and development

Lactic Acid

Lactic Acid is a chemical compound that is used in processed foods as a preservative, and as a curing agent, as well as a decontaminant during meat processing

Malic Acid

Malic Acid contributes to the sour flavor of fruits and is used as a food additive

Maltodextrin

Maltodextrin is a starch, used most often as a food additive in processed foods. It is produced through partial hydrolysis of the starch. It can have a sweet taste and is used as filler and a non-caking agent.

Modified Corn

Modified Corn is another name often used for Genetically Modified Corn

Modified Soy

Modified Soy is another name often used for Genetically Modified Soy.

Monosodium Glutomate

MSG, often called Glutamic Acid, is a naturally occurring non-essential Amino Acid. It is used to enhance other flavors in prepared foods.

It is used in a number of food additives including hydrolyzed vegetable protein and hydrolyzed yeast, and is often labeled in prepared foods as a "Natural Flavor". A food can be labeled with No MSG or No MSG added and still contains Glutamate

Natural Flavor

See Monosodium Glutamate

Pectins

Pectins are extracted from citrus fruits and are used as a gelling agent in jams and jellies, as a stabilizer agent in fruit juices and other foods

Potassium Chloride

Once known as Muriate of Potash, Potassium Chloride is often used as a fertilizer, but, it can be used intravenously to replenish electrolytes.

CAUTION: Large doses can slow or stop the heart. A lethal dose is estimated at 2.5-grams/kg-body weight for a healthy person.

Salmonella and Cooking Meats

Salmonella is a bacterium that exists in almost all animals. Usually, it is destroyed by freezing meats or even by heating the meat using ultra-violet or regular cooking methods for a minimum period of time.

You should always cook meats until the center of the meat reaches; (1) a temperature over 55C or 131F for at least 90 minutes, (2) 60C or 140F for at least 12 minutes or the most recommended temperature of all, 75C or 161F for at least 10 minutes.

Sodium Ascorbate

Sodium Ascorbate is a mineral salt of ascorbic acid (Vitamin C) and is an antioxidant that is used to control acidity. It can reduce hypertension and even help fight heart attacks in some people, and it has what are called **cytotoxic** effects on some malignant cells such as Melanomas.

It's well tolerated by most people, but it can cause; abdominal cramps, nausea and vomiting and some people can be allergic to it, with symptoms like; dizziness, itching, swelling, and even difficulty in breathing.

Sodium Phosphate

Sodium Phosphates are salts that are often used in the food industry as a leavening agent and to manage the pH level of processed foods. It can be used medically to control constipation and as an oral preparation before a colonoscopy.

NOTE: The medical uses of oral phosphates have been stopped in the US

Sucrose

Sucrose is a chemical compound generally known as table sugar

Syrup

Syrup is a combination of sugar and water that has been thickened over heat.

Table-B1-1 - Planting Times for Common Foods

Vegetable	Days to Maturity	Soil Temp for Germination (F)
• Beans; Bush, Pole	• 50 - 60	• 48-50
• Beets	• 55 - 65	• 39-41
• Broccoli	• 60 - 80	• 55-75
• Cabbage	• 80 - 110	• 38-40
• Cantaloupe	• 80 - 90	• 65-75
• Carrot	• 70 - 85	• 39-41
• Cauliflower	• 60 - 70	• 65-75
• Collards	• 55 - 75	• 40-50
• Corn; All	• 70 -90	• 45-50
• Cucumber	• 50 - 65	• 65-70
• Eggplant	• 75 - 85	• 40-45
• Kale	• 50 - 65	• 39-45
• Lettuce	• 65 - 85	• 40-75
• Mustard Greens	• 40 - 50	• 39-45
• Onion, Green	• 70 - 90	• 34-36
• Onion, Bulb	• 100 - 120	• 34-36
• Peas	• 60 - 70	• 34-36
• Pepper, Bell, Hot, Sweet	• 70 - 90	• 70-80
• Potato, Red, White	• 70 - 90	• 55-70
• Pumpkin	• 90 - 120	• 55-60
• Radish	• 25 - 30	• 39-41
• Spinach	• 40 - 45	• 55-65
• Squash, Summer	• 45 - 55	• 55-60
• Squash, Winter	• 90 - 120	• 55-60
• Tomato	• 70 - 90	• 50-55
• Turnip	• 45 - 60	• 55-60
• Watermelon	• 80 - 90	• 90-95

Table-B1-2 – FOOD Labeling – the GOOD and the Questionable

These are just a few of the more common food and product labels used today by the food industry. Others are being considered and hopefully our government will provide more and more stringent conditions for not only what is in our foods, but also what the big corporations are telling us.

Some of these are labeled as GOOD while some are just provided here as being informational and can be of questionable use to the public.

ANTIBACTERIAL – This label is very controversial and may eventually be banned or at least re-defined by the FDA in the near future. This claim for soaps and Cleaners has been questioned and some even recommend that the chemicals used be stopped because of their interference with some antibiotic medications.

CRUELTY FREE - This label is actually considered by many to be unregulated but some companies use 3rd-party companies to certify their manufacturing processes as being Cruelty Free in their use of animals. Animal Activists are especially critical of the use of this label, when the companies are using animals for product testing and can still get certified to use the label.

DOLPHIN SAFE - GOOD – This regulated label indicates that the fishing company does not use Purse Seine Nets and that it takes precautions to avoid trapping or catching Dolphins in their fishing nets.

FAIR TRADE - GOOD – This is a regulated label and certification is managed by FLO and FLO-CERT organizations. For a product to be labeled FAIRTRADE, at least 20% of its mass must be from a Fair-trade product. Fair trade products must meet certain labor, pricing, environmental and product development standards set by the FLO.

FREE RANGE - The USDA manages the use of this label, but there are no set standards for the size of the range area, the quality of the range area, nor the amount of time allowed for animals to range freely. The USDA regulates this label for Chickens only while regulations of its use for Beef and Pork are still not defined.

GRAIN FED - This is a pending USDA label. It is supposed to mean that the animals were fed grasses and even forage, and not grains that were industrially produced. This will not indicate the absence of Antibiotics or Hormones.

GRAIN FINISHED for FLAVOR - This label does not have a real definition and it is not regulated. It is supposed to mean that the animal was penned and fed grains for some undefined period of time before its slaughter. This is typically done to fatten the animal and improve the fat marbling in the meat. But it does not indicate how this is done nor what it was fed for the other part of its life.

GREEN SEAL - GOOD – This is a regulated label that is regulated by a non-profit organization. It indicates that the products production is done in a way that; reduces pollution and minimizes impact to the environment. It is used on such items as; food packaging, hand soaps, household cleaners, personal care products and more.

HUMANE RAISED and HANDLED, CERTIFIED - GOOD – This label indicates that the meat included, from Beef, Dairy, and Sheep, were raised to defined humane standards in a clean environment and were fed without the use of antibiotics or growth hormones. Also, they were slaughtered to defined humane standards.

HYPO-ALLERGENIC - There are no established standards for this label and its use is totally unregulated. The term itself is defined as a product or animal that is less allergenic than its peers. It is used extensively by the cosmetics industry but it is scientifically unsupportable as a standard.

NATURAL - This label is supposed to mean that the food has no bio-engineered or genetically modified ingredients. Presently, even though the FDA is selectively notifying some companies of their error in labeling, they have not, yet set any defined standard for products to be labeled as "natural".

NON-TOXIC - There are no standards for a product to meet in order to carry one of the dozens of popular non-toxic labels in use. There is no regulating organization and no defined requirements on products. It is implied, by some companies, that it means the labeled product is less dangerous to a person's health or to the environment.

ORGANIC - GOOD - This is a regulated label is used for the Food and Cotton industries to certify that the product is free of antibiotics and hormones and was grown in an environment free of any questionable chemicals or synthetic pesticides.

Table-B2-1 – FORAGING for plants – The GOOD and the BAD

A few of the many wild plants that you can find when foraging are listed alphabetically below along with the edible parts and also the plants that you might find which are Toxic.

EDIBLE PLANTS:

AGAVE – The Leaves, Flowers and Pods are edible, raw or cooked.

AMARANTH - Flowers and buds can be eaten as well as the leaves and seeds. Always boil the flowers or buds first.

ARCTIC WILLOW - Insides of young shoots are edible in early spring

ARROW ROOT - Rootstock is edible, but boil first

BAEL FRUIT - Ripened Fruit is edible, ripens in December.

BAMBOO - Young Shoots are edible, but boil first.

BANANA - Ripe Fruits, flowers, young shoots and "heart" of plant are edible.

BEARBERRY - Fruits, raw or cooked, leaves make a nice tea.

BEECH NUTS - Eat the Sweet Kernel of the nut.

BLACKBERRY - Fruits and peeled young shoots are edible.

BLUEBERRY - Ripe Fruits are edible.

BURDOCK - Young leafy stalks and roots are edible if cooked.

CANNA LILY - Roots and young shoots can be chopped into a meal.

CATTAIL - Young shoots are edible raw or cooked.

CEREUS CACTUS - Fruits are edible.

CHICORY - Leaves are edible as salad, boil roots for a coffee substitute.

CHUFA - Young tubers are edible.

COCONUT - The large nut provides a meaty liner as well as fruit and milk that are all edible.

CRANBERRY - The tart berries are edible.

CROWBERRY - The fresh fruits are edible or they can be dried for later use.

CUIPO TREE - Cut the root and hold horizontal, clean one end, put into mouth and tilt up to get a potato flavored water.

DANDELION - Every part of the plant is edible, boil roots and eat flowers and leaves raw or cooked, pull leaves before the plant flowers for best taste.

DATE PALM - Eat the fruits fresh or dry them in the sun for later use.

DAYLILY - Eat green leaves, tubers and flowers raw or cooked

DEWBERRY - Fruits and peeled young shoots are edible

ELDERBERRY - Fruits and flowers are edible.

ESKIMO POTATO - Eat the tubers after boiling.

FILBERT NUT - The kernel of the nut is edible

FOXTAIL GRASS - The mature grains of the grass are edible but are best when boiled.

HUCKLEBERRY - Fruits and peeled young shoots are edible

INDIAN POTATO - Eat the tubers after boiling.

INDIAN STRAWBERRY - Fruit is edible raw.

HACKBERRY - Fallen berries are ripe and edible

HAZELNUT - The kernel of the nut is edible.

JUNIPER - The berries are edible raw or roasted, boil twigs in a tea.

LOTUS - The whole plant is edible, boil or bake the roots or leaves. Eat seeds or grind them into a meal.

MANGO - Eat the flesh raw or ripe, roast the seed kernels.

MARSH MARIGOLD - All parts are edible but boil before eating.

MILKWEED - Harvest the flowers and boil before eating

NETTLE - Wear gloves to harvest this plant, boil young shoots or leaves and eat.

OAK NUTS - Soak acorns for a couple of days to remove bitter taste and eat or grind into a flour.

ORACH - All parts are edible, chop into small pieces and boil.

OXEYE DAISY - Unopened buds and greens are edible and tasty. Use fresh green leaves in salads

PALMETTO PALM - Fruits and "heart" of Palm are edible. Grind seeds into flour.

PAPAYA - Fruits are edible raw or cooked.

PINE NUTS - The nuts are edible raw or dried and the inside of the twigs are edible.

PLANTAIN - Ripe fruits, flowers, young shoots and "heart" of the plant are edible.

POKEWEED - The leaves of young plants are edible if washed and boiled twice changing the water both times to remove the poisons. Poisonous if not washed and boiled at least twice.

PERSIMMON - Eat ripened raw fruit, unripe fruit is very sour, roasted seeds are good as are the raw leaves

PINCUSHION CACTUS - Cut open for the water inside.

PRICKLY PEAR - The plant and the peeled fruits are edible, roasted and ground seeds make a nice flour.

PURSLANE - The whole plant is edible raw. Wash and boil the leaves for a nice edible salad.

RASPBERRY - The ripe fruit is edible.

REED - The whole plant is edible raw or cooked as a salad.

REINDEER MOSS - The whole plant is edible, soak in water to soften the stalks.

ROCK TRIPE - The whole plant is edible, soak in several changes of water to remove some of the bitterness.

ROSE APPLE - The fruit is edible either raw or cooked

ROSE HIPS - Rose Hips are edible both raw and cooked.

SASSAFRAS - The plant has a unique root beer scent, the twigs and leaves are edible, the roots can be dried and boiled to make a nice tea.

SEA ROCKET - The plant is edible and the leaves make a tasty addition to fresh salads.

SHEEP SORREL - The whole plant is edible, raw or cooked.

SORGHUM - The young grains are edible raw, The plant is edible and the leaves make a tasty addition to fresh salads. Cook older plant grains, boil the stalks to make molasses.

STERCULIA - The seeds of the red pods have a cocoa flavor and can be eaten raw or roasted

SUGARCANE - Peel the outer layer of the stalk and eat the inside raw, or boil the stalks in water for a sweet beverage.

TAMARIND - The pulp around the seeds of the fruit is edible raw, the seeds should be cooked before consuming them

THISTLE - Peel the stalks and boil before eating them, roots can be boiled and eaten.

TREE FERN - Boil the young leaves and eat as greens.

WALNUT - The kernel of the walnut is edible and nutritious.

WATERCRESS - Snap off the leaves and flowers and add them to fresh salads or soups, as you would use chives.

WATER LILY - The flowers and seeds are edible raw or cooked.

WATER PLANTAIN - Boil the rootstock in water to remove bitterness.

WILD CRAB APPLE - Eat ripe fruits but do not eat the seeds.

WILD DOCK - Wash the leaves several times to weaken the flavor, and eat raw or lightly cooked.

WILD GOURD - Cook the green fruits, or eat the leaves, flowers, and young shoots after cooking them.

WILD GRAPE VINE - The fruits (grapes) are edible and nutritious.

WILD GARLIC - The bulbs are edible raw or cooked in soups and store well when dried

WILD LEEKS - The bulbs are edible either raw or cooked in soups. Leeks have a strong Garlic like flavor.

WILD ONION - The bulbs are edible raw or cooked in soups and the greens are good in salads.

WILD RICE - Peel the stems and roots to boil and eat, remove the rice from mature husks and boil or roast the rice.

WILD ROSE - Whether eaten raw or boiled, the flowers and the buds (or rose hips) are edible, and the leaves make a nice tea.

WILD SORREL - The whole plant is edible and is better if chopped up and boiled.

YAM BEAN - The turnip-like root is nutritious and flavorful with a nutty flavor.

YELLOW WATER LILY - Boil the peeled roots, seeds of the fruits can be roasted.

NOT EDIBLE PLANTS:

ANGELS TRUMPET - NOT EDIBLE - Causes paralysis of muscles, hallucinations and insanity

ANGEL WINGS - (Caladium) NOT EDIBLE – All Parts are TOXIC

AUTUMN CROCUS - NOT EDIBLE – All Parts are TOXIC

AZALEAS - NOT EDIBLE – All Parts are TOXIC

BITTERSWEET NIGHTSHADE - NOT EDIBLE – All Parts are TOXIC

BLACK NIGHTSHADE - NOT EDIBLE – All Parts are TOXIC

BLEEDING HEART - NOT EDIBLE – All Parts are TOXIC

BLISTER BUSH - NOT EDIBLE – All Parts are TOXIC

CALLA LILY - NOT EDIBLE – All Parts are TOXIC

CARDINAL FLOWER - NOT EDIBLE – Poisonous if eaten, can cause Depression, Exhaustion, or a comatose state

CARNATION - NOT EDIBLE – All Parts are TOXIC

CHRISTMAS ROSE - NOT EDIBLE – All Parts are TOXIC

COLUMBINE - NOT EDIBLE – All Parts are TOXIC

DAFFODILS - The FLOWERS are NOT TOXIC – The BULB is TOXIC

DELPHINIUM - NOT EDIBLE – All Parts are TOXIC

FIRE LILY - NOT EDIBLE – All Parts are TOXIC

FOXGLOVE - NOT EDIBLE – All Parts are TOXIC

GOLDEN CHAIN - NOT EDIBLE – All Parts are TOXIC

GOLDEN TRUMPET VINE - NOT EDIBLE – All Parts are TOXIC

HELIOTROPE - NOT EDIBLE – All Parts are TOXIC

JACK in the PULPIT - NOT EDIBLE – ROOTS are TOXIC

JAPANESE SPURGE - NOT EDIBLE – All Parts are TOXIC

LANTANA - NOT EDIBLE – All Parts are TOXIC

LILY of the VALLEY - NOT EDIBLE – All Parts are TOXIC

MONKSHOOD - NOT EDIBLE – All Parts are EXTREMELY TOXIC, will cause death

OLEANDER - NOT EDIBLE – Can cause Cardiac Arrest

PANSY - NOT EDIBLE – SEEDS are TOXIC

PEONY - NOT EDIBLE – ROOTS are TOXIC

PRIMROSE - NOT EDIBLE – All Parts are TOXIC

RAINBOW LEUCOTHOE - NOT EDIBLE – LeaVes and Nectar are TOXIC

ROUGH-LEAF HYDRANGEA - NOT EDIBLE – All Parts are TOXIC

STAR OF BETHLEHEM - NOT EDIBLE – All Parts are TOXIC

STRAWBERRY - The fruit is edible raw or cooked, but eat only the fruit from white-flowering plants. Plants with flowers that are not white can be poisonous.

WISTERIA - NOT EDIBLE – SEEDS and PODS are TOXIC

YELLOW OLEANDER - NOT EDIBLE - Highly Toxic, causes extreme burning in throat, delirium and if person falls into a coma death can follow.

Table-B2-2 – Major U.S GRADES for OLIVE OIL

Grade	Definition
Extra Virgin Olive Oil	Excellent flavor and Fatty acid content less than 0.8%
Virgin Olive Oil	Good flavor and Fatty acid content less than 2%
Virgin Olive Oil Not Fit For Human Consumption Without Further Processing	Poor flavor, mechanically extracted and equivalent to IOC's lampante oil.
Olive Oil	A mixture of both refined and virgin oils
Refined Olive Oil	An Oil that is made from refined Oils with some process restrictions.

DISCLAIMER

I have been told that there are more Lawyers in the US than in all of the other nations of the world, combined. So, at this point I need to add a disclaimer for my own protection. Although I have spent numerous hours researching the web and building this list of survival suggestions for you, I assume no responsibility for your interpretation or your use of what I have written here.

Nor do I assume any responsibility for any injury, harm or distress that you or anyone else may incur if you or they end up foraging, collecting, cooking, medicating, using or consuming anything or any idea based on what I have put together in this book. You should use this information as a reference of ideas for your own research.

SOURCES

The sources for the information provided here are varied and numerous. So much of what I have written is from my own experiences during my own life. I learned how to work on a farm by working on a farm. I learned how to hunt and fish and grow my own foods by doing these things myself. Of course, my Dad, my aunts and uncles and so many others taught me how to do so many seemingly simple things, that I now realize were true survival skills.

To paraphrase a favorite country song of mine;

I can skin a Deer, I can run a Trotline; and this Country Boy can Survive!

I learned so much just by listening to my family members who were farmers but also in this computer age we live in, by simply doing my own research on the web and learning the truth about processed foods, and the chemicals many corporations have been subjecting the world's population to. Such chemicals as antibiotics and hormones in beef and other meats, along with cancer and other disease causing chemicals that are used to increase production volumes and thus profits, are often used with a disdain for what they might be doing to consumers.

So you will not find a long list of individual sources such as you find in many technical manuals and reference sources. I checked and cross-checked what I have put into this book, as best I could. But, I can only tell you that most of what you read here is gleaned from a lifetime of experience and if you think it might be useful then you should perform your own "investigation" about anything that you might question, on the web and in libraries, and find out for yourselves. And the photography used is either my own, from government sites, or it was copied from Public Domain sites.

My name is Don Bobbitt and I Wrote this Book because

I WAS JUST WONDERING!

THE END

INDEX

A

214

www.ingramcontent.com/pod-product-compliance
Lightning Source LLC
Chambersburg PA
CBHW051738250726
48659CB00001B/122